Implantable Cardiac Pacemakers and Defibrillators: All You Wanted to Know

Implantable Cardiac Pacemakers and Defibrillators:
All You Wanted to Know

EDITED BY

Anthony W.C. Chow
The Heart Hospital
UCLH NHS Foundation Trust
London, UK

Alfred E. Buxton
Cardiovascular Division, Brown Medical School
Rhode Island Hospital
Providence, Rhode Island, USA

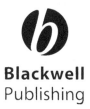

Blackwell
Publishing

© 2006 by Blackwell Publishing Ltd

BMJ Books is an imprint of the BMJ Publishing Group Limited, used under licence

Blackwell Publishing, Inc., 350 Main Street, Malden, Massachusetts 02148-5020, USA
Blackwell Publishing Ltd, 9600 Garsington Road, Oxford OX4 2DQ, UK
Blackwell Publishing Asia Pty Ltd, 550 Swanston Street, Carlton, Victoria 3053, Australia

The right of the Author to be identified as the Author of this Work has been
asserted in accordance with the Copyright, Designs and Patents Act 1988.

First published 2006

Library of Congress Cataloging-in-Publication Data

Implantable cardiac pacemakers and defibrillators : all you wanted to
know / edited by Anthony W.C. Chow and Alfred E. Buxton.
    p. ; cm.
Includes bibliographical references and index.
ISBN: 978-0-7279-1566-5 (pbk. : alk. paper)
    1. Cardiac pacing. 2. Electric countershock. I. Chow, Anthony
W.C. II. Buxton, Alfred E.
    [DNLM: 1. Cardiac Pacing, Artificial. 2. Defibrillators, Implantable.
3. Pacemaker, Artificial. WG 168 I34 2006]
RC684.P3I47 2006
617.4'120645–dc22

                                                                      2005022328

ISBN: 978-0-7279-1566-5

A catalogue record for this title is available from the British Library

Set in 9.5/12 pt Meridian by Newgen Imaging Systems (P) Ltd, Chennai, India

Commissioning Editor: Mary Banks
Development Editors: Veronica Pock and Elisabeth Dodds
Production Controller: Debbie Wyer

For further information on Blackwell Publishing, visit our website:
http://www.blackwellpublishing.com

The publisher's policy is to use permanent paper from mills that operate a sustainable
forestry policy, and which has been manufactured from pulp processed using acid-free
and elementary chlorine-free practices. Furthermore, the publisher ensures that the text
paper and cover board used have met acceptable environmental accreditation standards.

Contents

List of contributors

Editors

Anthony W.C. Chow, The Heart Hospital, UCLH NHS Foundation Trust, London, UK

Alfred E. Buxton, Cardiovascular Division, Brown Medical School, Rhode Island Hospital, Providence, Rhode Island, USA

Contributors

Alfred E. Buxton, Cardiovascular Division, Brown Medical School, Rhode Island Hospital, Providence, Rhode Island, USA

Henry F. Clemo, Department of Medicine, Medical College of Virginia, Richmond, Virginia, USA

Anthony W.C. Chow, The Heart Hospital, UCLH NHS Foundation Trust, London, UK

Martin R. Cowie, National Heart and Lung Institute, Imperial College, London, UK

D. Wyn Davies, Waller Department of Cardiology, St. Mary's Hospital, London, UK

Kenneth A. Ellenbogen, Department of Electrophysiology, Medical College of Virginia, Richmond, Virginia, USA

Malcolm Kirk, Department of Medicine, Brown Medical School, Providence, Rhode Island, USA

Kristin E. Ellison, Department of Medicine, Brown Medical School, Providence, Rhode Island, USA

Rebecca E. Lane, SpR Cardiology, London, UK

Martin Lowe, The Heart Hospital, London, UK

Nicholas S. Peters, Waller Department of Cardiology, St. Mary's Hospital, London, UK

Vias Markides, Waller Department of Cardiology, St. Mary's Hospital, London, UK

Richard Schilling, St. Bartholomew's Hospital and Queen Mary University of London, London, UK

Oliver R. Segal, Waller Department of Cardiology, St. Mary's Hospital, London, UK

Simon Sporton, St. Bartholomew's Hospital and Queen Mary University of London, London, UK

Aneesh V. Tolat, Beth Israel-Deaconness Medical Center, Boston, Massachusetts, USA

Mark Turner, Royal Bristol Infirmary, London, UK

Fiona Walker, University College London Hospitals NHS Trust, The Heart Hospital, London, UK

Peter J. Zimetbaum, Beth Israel-Deaconness Medical Center, Boston, Massachusetts, USA

Introduction

Advances in pacing and defibrillator technology in recent years, supported by findings of a large number of well-designed, randomized clinical trials have resulted in the increasing application of this technology for the treatment of a variety of cardiac disorders. The result has been a huge increase in the numbers of devices implanted for tachyarrhythmias and bradyarrhythmias, as well as heart failure therapy. As newer implantable devices have acquired increasing functionality, interpretation of their operation has become progressively complex.

This book is intended as an introduction for all medical and allied professionals including cardiovascular trainees, generalists, nonpacing specialists, and associated medical personnel, who want to understand and embrace this expanding field.

Our aim with this book is to remove some of the mystique surrounding pacemakers and defibrillators, taking the reader from basic concepts to complex functions of these devices, covering the indications for their use and common problems encountered with this technology, in a logical, evidence-based manner. We have also taken a "how-to-do-it" approach for certain areas of implantable device function. The inclusion of these sections will be of interest for trainees and those who do not normally deal with the technical aspect of the discipline. This type of information is often difficult to acquire, and normally learned at the bedside, or in the clinical electrophysiology laboratory.

To many, implantable pacemakers and defibrillators appear as unfathomable black boxes. These devices are in fact pieces of hardware that function with intrinsic logic. It is an introduction to these concepts that we seek to convey with this book. We have brought together here a group of authors who have gone to extraordinary lengths in order to demystify the function of pacemakers, implantable defibrillators, and cardiac resynchronization devices with the hope of improving the readers' understanding of these arrhythmia devices and their functions.

It should be recognized by all that this field is moving rapidly, as a result of both technological advances as well as clinical data derived from clinical trials. Nevertheless, we anticipate that the fundamental principles underlying pacemaker and defibrillator function outlined herein will remain valid for the foreseeable future.

Anthony W.C. Chow and Alfred E. Buxton

CHAPTER 1

Basic principles of pacing

Malcolm Kirk

The aim of this chapter is to give sufficient background and information about cardiac pacemakers to allow interpretation of electrocardiograms (ECGs) and telemetry strips of normal pacemaker behavior. For more in-depth inform-ation, such as would be necessary for programming pacemakers, a standard pacing text should be consulted. Several of these are listed in the bibliography. Most italicized terms are defined in the glossary at the end of the chapter.

Anatomy

The pertinent anatomy for cardiac pacing includes the sinoatrial (SA) node, the atrioventricular (AV) node, and the His-Purkinje system (Figure 1.1).

The SA node is located at the superior aspect of the *crista terminalis* (not pictured), near the junction with the superior vena cava. It is normally the dominant pacemaker in the heart, because its rate of depolarization exceeds that of other areas that normally possess properties of automaticity, such as the more inferior areas of the *crista terminalis* and the His-Purkinje system. The SA node can, in turn, be suppressed by an even faster rhythm, such as an atrial tachycardia, or pacing by an implanted pacemaker.

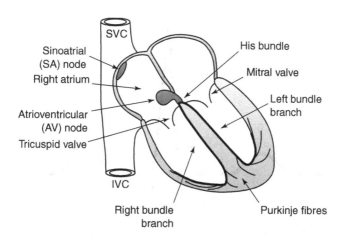

Figure 1.1 Schematic of conduction system anatomy

The AV node is normally the only electrical connection between the atria and the ventricles. Electrical activation proceeds from the right atrium, through the AV node to the His-Purkinje system, and then to the ventricles.

The His-Purkinje system comprises myocardial cells that are specialized for rapid conduction. Its anatomic components are (in order of activation) the His bundle, the bundle branches (right and left) and the Purkinje fibers. The His-Purkinje system delivers the electrical impulse rapidly from the AV node to widely dispersed areas of the left and right ventricular endocardium, making activation nearly simultaneous throughout the ventricles. This rapid conduction, and simultaneous activation of the right and left ventricles, results in the narrow QRS complex seen on a normal ECG. If an impulse is transmitted throughout the ventricle without using the His-Purkinje system, it takes longer for the ventricles to be activated, and hence the QRS complex is wider. An example would be a premature ventricular contraction (PVC). Another would be ventricular pacing, because the pacemaker lead is usually not positioned so as to activate initially the His-Purkinje system. (Furthermore, in this case the ventricles are activated sequentially rather than simultaneously.)

The components of the surface ECG reflect the cardiac chambers and conducting system (Figure 1.2). The activation of the atria creates the *P wave* on the surface ECG. Electrical conduction through the AV node to the His-Purkinje system is relatively slow, so there is normally a 120–200 millisecond (ms) delay between the start of atrial activation and the start of ventricular activation. The delay between the onset of the surface P wave and the onset of the QRS complex is due mostly to conduction through the AV node, with some contribution from intraatrial conduction, and His-Purkinje system conduction. The activation of the ventricles creates the QRS complex.

As noted above, the AV node and His-Purkinje system are normally the only electrical connection between the atria and the ventricles. Failure of electrical conduction through the AV node and/or His-Purkinje system results

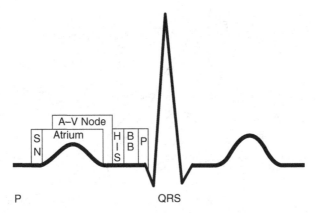

Figure 1.2 The conducting system is reflected in the normal QRS complex. SN = sinus node, His = His bundle, BB = bundle branches, P = Purkinje fibers.

in *heart block*, also known as AV block, and is one of the indications for pacemaker implantation (see Chapter 3). When assessing a pacemaker patient, it is important to consider whether or not the patient has intact *intrinsic conduction* through the AV node and His-Purkinje system. If electrical conduction from the atrium to the ventricles is not present (AV block), then the patient is likely to be dependent on ventricular pacing to maintain an adequate heart rate.

Physiology

Cardiac muscle cells, like other excitable cells, have a resting electrical gradient across the cell membrane. In the quiescent state (during diastole), the inside of the cell (cytoplasm) is electrically negative relative to the outside of the cell. That is to say, the cell membrane separates positive (outside) and negative (inside) charges. Thus the cell membrane is *polarized*. It becomes *depolarized* when an electrical current causes opening of sodium (Na^+) and calcium (Ca^{2+}) channels in the cell membrane, allowing these positive ions to rush into the cell. This flow of positive ions into the cell has two important consequences: propagation of electrical activity (the action potential) and contraction of the cell.

Propagation of the action potential
Propagation is the spread of depolarization in a wave across the heart. Because the flow of positive ions into the cell is itself a small current, it causes opening of Na^+ and Ca^{2+} channels in adjacent cells. The opening of these channels, in turn, creates a current that causes opening of channels in cells beyond, and so forth, so long as adjacent cells are *excitable*, and not *refractory* (see below).

Refractoriness
Refractoriness is a normal property of cardiac tissue. After depolarization, cells need a certain amount of time to recover before they can be stimulated again. In the most general sense, *refractoriness* is the opposite of *excitability*. After a cardiac muscle cell has been *depolarized* (also called *excited*), it cannot be depolarized again until the membrane has become polarized again (or repolarized). The time between an electrical stimulus that excites a certain part of the heart, and the latest repeat stimulus that cannot excite the same tissue is known as the *refractory period*. A stimulus that fails to excite the heart because it occurs too soon after the previous stimulus or depolarization is said to find the tissue *refractory*.

The amount of time required for recovery of excitability (i.e. the refractory period) depends on the type of cardiac tissue (atrium, ventricle, AV node, conducting system), and may be influenced by medications or by rate of stimulation. The refractory period of the AV node is important in pacing and atrial arrhythmias. It will determine how frequently atrial impulses can be transmitted to the ventricle. For example, in atrial fibrillation, the atrial rate can exceed 400 beats per minute (bpm), but not every impulse is transmitted to the ventricle. Most of the atrial beats will be blocked at the AV node, because they reached the AV node at a time when it is refractory and cannot conduct. The response of the AV node to rapid stimulation rates differs from other cardiac tissue, in that the refractory period of the AV node generally increases with increased rates of stimulation, whereas the refractory period of the atria and ventricles decreases with increased rates of stimulation. The AV node thus limits the maximum rate at which the ventricle can follow a rapid atrial rhythm.

Parts of a pacemaker system

A pacemaker consists of a *pulse generator* (Figure 1.3) and pacing *leads*.

The pulse generator contains the battery of the pacemaker, as well as the circuits that deliver the pacing stimuli. The lead input and circuitry in a pacemaker pulse generator dedicated to a particular chamber of the heart is known as a *channel*. For example, the ventricular channel transmits the ventricular pacing impulse to the ventricular lead.

Pacemaker leads are electrical conductors (wires), covered with insulation. They transmit the electrical impulses from the pulse generator to the heart, and from the heart to the pulse generator.

Pacemaker leads are usually inserted into the subclavian vein or its tributaries, and positioned on the inner surface (endocardium) of the heart. They are attached to the endocardium by a small screw mechanism, or are held in place by tines. If a screw (also known as a helix) is used to fix the lead to the heart, the lead is called an active fixation lead (Figure 1.4). A passive fixation

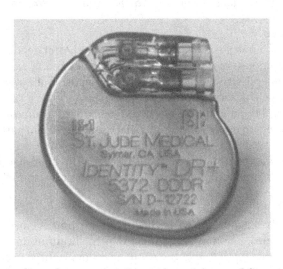

Figure 1.3 Pacemaker pulse generator. Dimensions: 4.4 cm × 5.2 cm × 0.6 cm. Courtesy of St. Jude Medical.

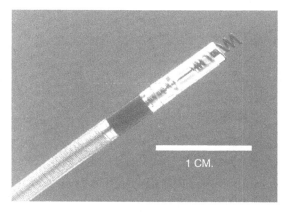

Figure 1.4 Active fixation lead. Courtesy of St. Jude Medical.

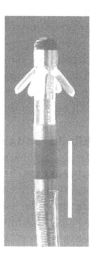

Figure 1.5 Passive fixation lead. The white bar is 1 Cm. Courtesy of St. Jude Medical.

lead has tines (Figure 1.5), which are designed to engage the trabeculae on the inner surface of the heart.

Pacemaker leads may also be placed on the outside of the heart (epicardium) during a surgical procedure. These leads are either sewn onto the heart, or fixed in place with a small screw-in mechanism.

The pacing stimulus

Pacemakers function by delivering a small electrical current to myocardial cells. The electrical activation spreads from cell to cell, throughout the heart. As each cell is electrically activated, it contracts.

The pacemaker delivers the electrical current between two points, called electrodes. These two points may be either two electrodes on the pacemaker lead, or one electrode on the pacemaker lead, and the metal covering of the

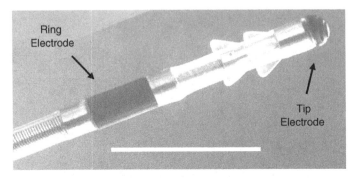

Figure 1.6 The two electrodes of a bipolar pacing lead. The white bar is 1 cm. Courtesy of St. Jude Medical.

pacemaker pulse generator. Electrical current is caused by the flow of electrons. This must occur in a circuit (i.e. a closed loop). A source of current, such as the battery of a pacemaker, will have a negative end (from which electrons are emitted) and a positive end (to which electrons are attracted). For reasons beyond the scope of this chapter, pacing is more efficient when the tip electrode of the pacing lead is the negative pole. The positive pole can either be a metallic ring, about a centimeter back from the tip of the lead (Figure 1.6), or can be the body of the pacemaker pulse generator itself.

Bipolar and unipolar pacing – ECG

Bipolar and *unipolar pacing* have different appearances on surface ECGs. If the current flows between the two electrodes on the pacemaker lead (the tip and the ring), this is referred to as bipolar pacing. If the current flows between the tip of the lead and the pacemaker generator, this is referred to as unipolar pacing. In unipolar pacing, the current travels through a large area of the body between the tip of the lead and the pulse generator. Unipolar pacing, therefore, creates a large *stimulus artifact* on the surface ECG. It may stimulate electrically excitable tissue, other than the heart, which lies in the path of the current. An example of such a tissue would be the pectoralis muscle over which the pacemaker generator is placed. The bipolar pacing stimulus may be very difficult to see on the surface ECG, because in bipolar pacing the distance between the two poles that deliver current (i.e. the tip and the ring of the pacemaker lead) is very small (about a centimeter), as illustrated in Figure 1.6. It will also be noted that leads that are used for bipolar pacing must have two insulated wires within its outer insulation: one wire for the negative pole (the tip), and one for the positive pole (the ring).

Pacing by defibrillators

The implantable cardioverter-defibrillator (usually called an ICD or defibrillator) was developed to detect life-threatening ventricular tachyarrhythmias,

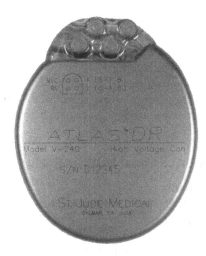

Figure 1.7 Defibrillator pulse generator.
Dimensions: 6.7 cm × 5.0 cm × 1.4 cm.
Courtesy of St. Jude Medical.

and terminate them by delivering a high-energy defibrillating shock to the heart. The pulse generator is somewhat larger than that of a pacemaker (Figure 1.7). All modern defibrillators also function as pacemakers. This is not commonly understood. A patient will often be told that he or she has "a pacemaker and a defibrillator" when the patient, in fact, has only a single device – a defibrillator. Modern defibrillators include nearly as many pacing features as modern pacemakers; anything in this chapter about pacemakers also applies to the pacing function of defibrillators, unless otherwise stated.

Single and dual chamber pacing

The word *chamber* in dual or single chamber pacing refers to a chamber of the heart in which a lead is placed. Each lead is connected to a *channel* of the pacemaker (see section on "Parts of a pacemaker system"). The channel is the part of the pacemaker circuitry and memory assigned to that particular lead (and therefore, the corresponding cardiac chamber).

A single chamber pacemaker usually has a pacing lead in either the right atrium, or the right ventricle. These would be called, respectively, an atrial single chamber pacemaker and a ventricular single chamber pacemaker. (They are also sometimes called an AAI pacemaker and a VVI pacemaker, respectively, for reasons that will become apparent in the section on "Pacing modes.")

A standard dual chamber pacemaker has a lead in the right atrium and a lead in the right ventricle. (A dual chamber defibrillator has a pacing lead in the right atrium and a pacing/defibrillation lead in the right ventricle. The latter delivers the defibrillation shock, as well as pacing.) Biventricular pacing is a newly developed type of pacing incorporating a third lead, which is positioned to activate the posterolateral wall of the left ventricle. This results in "ventricular resynchronization," which can improve ventricular hemodynamics, and relieve heart failure symptoms in certain patients with heart failure and conduction abnormalities. (This is detailed in Chapter 7.)

The interaction between the atrial and ventricular chambers in dual chamber pacing can be somewhat complex. Failure to understand this interaction is the source of many questions about pacemaker behavior. The elements needed to understand dual chamber pacing are covered below.

Conceptual building blocks of pacemaker function

Pacing

Pacing refers to the regular output of electrical current, for the purpose of depolarizing the cardiac tissue in the immediate vicinity of the lead, with resulting propagation of a wave of depolarization throughout that chamber. A pacemaker will pace at a certain frequency, or rate, for example, 60 bpm. This rate is *programmable*. That is, it can be changed by using the manufacturer's *programmer*.

Sensing

The heart's intrinsic electrical activity (i.e. the P wave or QRS complex) transmits a small electrical current (a few millivolts), through the pacemaker leads, to the pulse generator. This current can be registered or *sensed* by the pacemaker circuitry. Pacemaker sensing describes the response of a pacemaker to intrinsic heartbeats. The P waves, or atrial activity, are transmitted through the atrial lead (if present) to the atrial channel of the pacemaker, and sensed as atrial activity. Ventricular activity (the QRS complex) is transmitted through the ventricular lead (if present) to the ventricular channel of the pacemaker, and this is sensed as ventricular activity.

For electrical activity to be transmitted from the heart to the pacemaker, a closed electrical circuit must be present, just the same as for an electrical impulse to be transmitted from the pacemaker to the heart. Thus, just as with pacing, sensing can be unipolar or bipolar. *Bipolar sensing* detects the intrinsic electrical activity occurring between the tip electrode and the ring electrode of the lead. *Unipolar sensing* detects electrical activity occurring between the tip of the lead, and the metal shell of the pulse generator. Because this is a much larger area, other electrical signals, such as might be generated by the muscles of the diaphragm or sources outside the body, are more likely to be detected (and therefore incorrectly interpreted by the pacemaker as heart beats).

It is important to note that the only way the pacemaker can determine which chamber a signal originates from is by which lead transmits the signal to the pacemaker. For example, the pacemaker will interpret any electrical signal transmitted through the atrial lead to the atrial channel as a P wave, even if the signal is in fact a QRS complex large enough in amplitude to be sensed by the atrial channel.

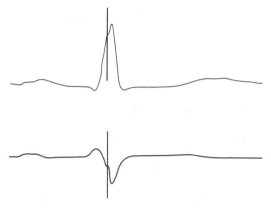

Figure 1.8 A single P–QRS complex is seen in two leads in a patient with a pacemaker. The vertical black line marks the instant when the pacemaker *senses* the QRS complex. Note that sensing by the pacemaker occurs well after the onset of the surface QRS. Up until this point, the pacemaker is not "aware" that a QRS complex is in progress. This illustrates how a normally functioning pacemaker can deliver a pacing spike early in the QRS complex, before it senses the presence of that complex.

Note also that the time at which the pacemaker senses the atrial or ventricular signal is not necessarily the beginning of the P wave or QRS. The pacemaker cannot sense activity in a chamber until the electrical activity actually reaches the pacemaker lead. Figure 1.8 illustrates that sensing in the ventricle occurs after the onset of the QRS complex.

Inhibition of output

A pacemaker can be programmed to inhibit pacing if it senses intrinsic activity, or it can be programmed to ignore intrinsic activity and deliver a pacing stimulus anyway. If a pacemaker is set so that it can be inhibited by *intrinsic beats*, then the pacemaker will not deliver a stimulus if it senses an intrinsic beat at the proper time. For example, if a pacemaker is set to pace in this way at 60 bpm, it will deliver a pacing stimulus only if an intrinsic beat does not occur within 1 second of the last sensed or *paced beat*.

Triggered pacing

Pacemakers can be programmed to deliver a pacing stimulus whenever intrinsic activity is sensed. This type of pacing is most often used in dual chamber pacemakers. Dual chamber pacemakers can be programmed to sense activity in one chamber (usually the atrium) and deliver a pacing stimulus in the other chamber (usually the ventricle) after a certain time delay. This is known as triggered pacing. When referring to the appearance of this type of pacing on telemetry or ECGs, it is commonly said that the ventricle is *tracking* the atrium, because if the atrial rate becomes faster, the ventricular pacing rate will follow faster, in a 1 : 1 relationship. Thus the exact rate of ventricular pacing will not be determined by any *setting* on the pacemaker, but by the

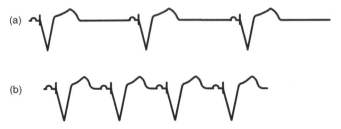

Figure 1.9 Triggered pacing. (a) and (b) both show atrial sensing, and ventricular pacing, in a tracking mode. The pacemaker settings are the same in both panels. The difference is that in (b) the intrinsic atrial rate is faster.

patient's own atrial rate (Figure 1.9). One would want to limit, of course, the maximum rate at which the pacemaker will track the atrial rhythm with ventricular pacing. This is discussed more extensively in the section on "Basic pacemaker programming – timing cycles."

Pacing modes

A standard pacemaker code has been developed jointly by the North American Society for Pacing and Electrophysiology, and the British Pacing and Electrophysiology Group (the NASPE/BPEG Generic Code, known as the NBG Code). The pacing function provided by a pacemaker (or defibrillator) is usually given by a series of three or four letters. (There is a fifth position in the code, which is not commonly used.) Each position denotes a different aspect of pacemaker function. The identity of the letter in that position specifies the function. A given combination of three or four letters is called a *mode*. A more in-depth discussion of these modes, and in the clinical scenarios for which each is used, appears in Chapter 3.

The positions and letters are as follows:
- Position 1: chamber being paced

    V = ventricle
    A = atrium
    D = atrium and ventricle (dual)
    O = no pacing.

- Position 2: chamber being sensed

    V = ventricle
    A = atrium
    D = atrium and ventricle (dual)
    O = no sensing.

- Position 3: pacing response to a *sensed beat*

    I = inhibited
    T = triggered

D = inhibited or triggered (dual) depending on the chamber
O = neither inhibited or triggered.

- Position 4: rate response or absence thereof (see section on "Basic pacemaker programming – sensing, pacing , and refractory periods")

    R = rate responsive
    O = absence of rate response. (But this is usually just omitted.)

Here are some examples:
- The VVI mode paces and senses only in the ventricle.

    Position 1 – V indicates that it will pace only in the ventricle.
    Position 2 – V indicates that it senses intrinsic heartbeats only in the ventricle.
    Position 3 – I indicates that the response to a sensed heartbeat is inhibition of ventricular pacing.
    Position 4 – blank, indicating that it is not rate responsive.

- The VAT mode would pace as follows:

    Position 1 – V indicates that it will pace only in the ventricle.
    Position 2 – A indicates that it will sense only in the atrium.
    Position 3 – T indicates that the pacemaker will deliver a ventricular stimulus every time it senses an atrial beat.
    Position 4 – blank, indicating that it is not rate responsive.

- DDD is a common mode. It operates as follows:

    Position 1 – D indicates that the pacemaker will pace in both the atrium and ventricle.
    Position 2 – D indicates that it will sense in both the atrium and the ventricle.
    Position 3 – D indicates that it will respond to a sensed beat in either chamber with inhibition of pacing output in that chamber, but it will also deliver a pacing stimulus in the ventricle after an atrial beat is sensed, unless there is inhibition by an intrinsic ventricular beat (i.e. triggered response).
    Position 4 – blank, indicating that it is not rate responsive.

Therefore, depending on the patient's intrinsic heart rate, and the programmed settings, a pacemaker in DDD mode might pace both the atrium and the ventricle, pace neither (sense in both), pace the atrium with intrinsic conduction to the ventricle (ventricular pacing output inhibited by sensed *R waves*) or track intrinsic P waves with ventricular pacing. These are illustrated in Figure 1.10.

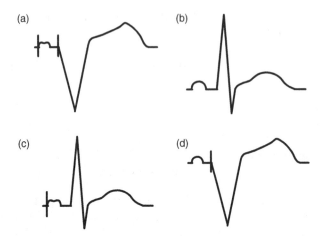

Figure 1.10 Types of pacing and sensing possible in DDD mode. (a) Pacing both the atrium and the ventricle; (b) pacing neither (sensing in both); (c) pacing the atrium with intrinsic conduction to the ventricle (ventricular pacing output inhibited by sensed R waves); (d) tracking intrinsic P waves with ventricular pacing. Note that which of these four electrograms is seen depends on the relationship of the intrinsic atrial rate and PR interval to the pacemaker lower rate and AV delay settings.

VOO is the simplest pacing mode (Figure 1.11).

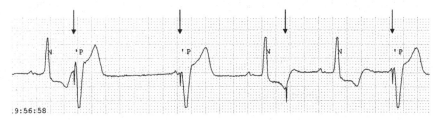

Figure 1.11 VOO pacing. The pacemaker is set in VOO mode. This is known as an *asynchronous* mode because the pacing stimuli are unrelated to the intrinsic rhythm. The arrows indicate the pacing stimuli, which are delivered at a rate of 40 bpm, and fall in random relationship to the intrinsic rhythm. Note that the first pacing stimulus falls just after an intrinsic QRS. It is not inhibited by the preceding QRS, which is not sensed because there is no sensing in this mode (the second position in the code is "O"). The third pacing stimulus falls when the ventricle is *refractory*, and so it fails to *capture* (i.e. it does not result in a QRS complex). The "N" and "P" are drawn in by the telemetry system when it designates beats as normal and paced, respectively.

Position 1 – V indicates that the pacemaker paces only in the ventricle.
Position 2 – O indicates that the pacemaker does not sense intrinsic activity; therefore, the third letter must also be O because it cannot have any response to intrinsic activity.
Position 3 – O indicates it is neither triggered nor inhibited by sensed activity.
Position 4 – blank, indicating that it is not rate responsive.

Basic pacemaker programming – sensing, pacing, and refractory periods

Sensing and pacing

The amount of electrical current delivered by a pacemaker is adjustable. The minimum amount of energy required to pace the heart can be found by decreasing the output energy until the pacing stimulus no longer causes depolarization of the atria or ventricles, seen as a P wave or QRS complex following the pacing stimulus artifact. The minimum energy needed to pace is called the pacing threshold. The output is set sufficiently above this threshold (often twice the threshold) to provide a safety margin for pacing *capture*, without excessive battery drain.

Sensing is conceptually more difficult. In order not to pace the heart inappropriately, the pacemaker must be able to sense intrinsic local depolarization. The *sensitivity* of a pacemaker channel is the threshold that the intrinsic electrical activity transmitted from that chamber must meet to be registered by the pacemaker. For example, if ventricular sensing is set to 2.5 mV, then the amplitude of the intrinsic QRS complex, as transmitted by the ventricular pacing lead to the pacemaker, must be at least 2.5 mV for the pacemaker to register that an intrinsic QRS complex has occurred. This is illustrated in Figure 1.12. Increasing the sensitivity value raises the threshold that the intrinsic activity must meet to be registered (i.e. it makes the pacemaker less sensitive). Proper adjustment of this level for an individual patient allows sensing of intrinsic activity without *oversensing* of extraneous activity, such as T waves, muscle potentials from the diaphragm, or sensing of R waves on the atrial lead.

Rate response

Currently available pacemakers (and defibrillators) can be programmed to vary the pacing rate in response to the patient's level of activity. Various

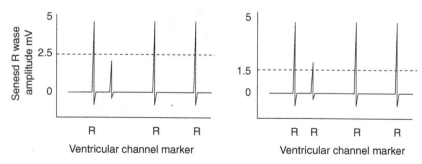

Figure 1.12 The second intrinsic complex (a PVC) does not create a large enough signal to be sensed in the ventricular channel with the sensing set at 2.5 mV (dotted line). Therefore, the pacemaker does not recognize the presence of the second intrinsic R wave. (The marker channel at the bottom indicates which intrinsic R waves are sensed by the pacemaker.) If the sensitivity (i.e. the threshold for sensing) had been lowered to 1.5 mV, the second beat would have been sensed.

types of sensors have been developed to allow the pacemaker to sense the patient's level of activity. The parameters sensed include patient movement, respiration, and changes in the T wave. Activation of the sensor by changes in these factors, which are not related to exercise, might be a cause of more rapid than expected pacing at rest. For example, hyperventilation or an activity that causes motion of the pacemaker pulse generator (e.g. physical therapy of the chest or shoulder) may increase the activity of pacemakers driven by minute ventilation and accelerometer sensors, respectively.

Refractory period

Pacemakers have refractory periods on each channel, which are generally programmable. During the refractory periods, sensed events are ignored. The most clinically important refractory period occurs in dual chamber pacing. It is the *postventricular atrial refractory period*, or *PVARP*. This is the period after a ventricular sensed or paced event, when the atrial channel is refractory. The effect is that in a dual chamber tracking mode, a P wave that falls shortly after the QRS complex (either a paced or intrinsic QRS) will not be *tracked*. That is, it will not be followed by a ventricular paced event. An important function of PVARP is to prevent pacemaker-mediated tachycardia. Pacemaker-mediated tachycardia (often abbreviated: "PMT") begins when a ventricular sensed or

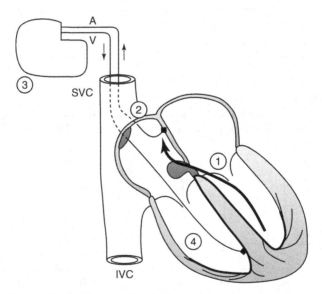

Figure 1.13 Pacemaker-mediated tachycardia. Step 1: conduction retrogradely from the ventricles to the right atrium through the AV node. Step 2: sensing of the resulting retrograde P wave by the atrial channel of the pacemaker. Step 3: triggered ventricular pacing tracking the sensed atrial event. (Note that the pacemaker will deliver ventricular pacing no faster than the upper tracking rate.) The paced ventricular beat is again conducted retrogradely up the His-Purkinje system, beginning step 1 again.

paced beat is transmitted *retrogradely* (from ventricle to atrium) through the His-Purkinje system and AV node, resulting in atrial activation. Without a pacemaker, the resulting P wave would not be conducted back to the ventricle, because the AV node and His-Purkinje system are *refractory*, having just been activated retrogradely. However, if the patient has a dual chamber pacemaker set in the tracking mode, then the pacemaker can sense the resulting P wave, and "track" it by delivering a ventricular impulse after an appropriate delay. Thus an endless loop is created. The electrical activity is transmitted from the ventricle to the atrium through the His-Purkinje system and AV node, and from the atrium to the ventricle through the pacemaker (Figure 1.13). The rate of PMT will be limited by the upper rate limit of the pacemaker (see section on "Basic pacemaker programming – timing cycles"), because the pacemaker will not track atrial beats faster than this rate. The presence of a PVARP helps prevent PMT. If atrial beats that have been transmitted retrogradely from the ventricle fall within the PVARP, then the pacemaker will not track them and they will not be transmitted back to the ventricle via ventricular pacing.

The PVARP also allows the pacemaker to respond to fast atrial rates in a physiologic fashion (see section on Upper rate behavior). The PVARP thus partially mimics the normal physiology of the intrinsic conduction system (see discussion of AV node refractory period in the section on "Physiology").

Basic pacemaker programming – timing cycles

The lower rate limit

This is the simplest aspect of pacemaker timing. In AOO or VOO (*asynchronous*) mode, this is the rate at which the pacemaker will pace. In AAI, or VVI mode, this is the rate at which the pacemaker will pace, unless it is inhibited by intrinsic beats occurring at a faster rate. (Two reasons that the heart rate may fall below the lower rate limit of the pacemaker are hysteresis and sleep function, both described below in the FAQ section.) If the pacer is in a rate-responsive (or rate-modulated) mode, then the actual lower rate limit will vary, depending on the activity of the rate-response sensor, but will not be less than the programmed lower rate limit.

AV delay

The AV delay is the time interval between an atrial paced or sensed event, and the delivery of a ventricular pacing stimulus. Because it involves events in two chambers, it is a programmable parameter in dual chamber pacemakers, but is not found in single chamber pacemakers. It is analogous to the intrinsic PR interval, in that it allows time for atrial contraction, and active ventricular filling, before ventricular contraction occurs. There are two types of AV delay: *sensed AV delay* and *paced AV delay*. The terms "sensed" and "paced" refer to events in the atrium.

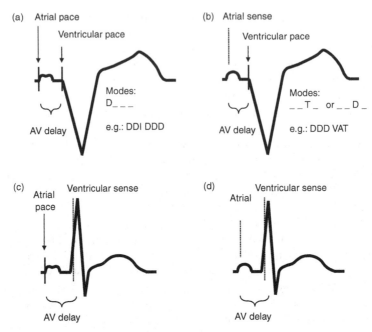

Figure 1.14 AV delay. (a) and (c) Paced AV delay in a dual chamber pacing mode. (b) and (d) Sensed AV delay in a triggered mode. The AV delay is a programmed parameter. (a) and (b) show a programmed AV delay that is shorter than intrinsic conduction. The pacer delivers a pacing stimulus at the end of the AV delay. In (c) and (d) a longer AV delay is programmed. An intrinsic QRS is sensed before the end of the AV delay, and ventricular pacing is inhibited. Note that bottom panels illustrate modes with ventricular sensing.

Paced AV delay
This is the delay (Figure 1.14a) between the delivery of the atrial pacing stimulus, and the delivery of the ventricular pacing stimulus. It therefore occurs in modes in which both chambers are paced. Examples would be DDD mode, DDI mode, and DOO mode.

Sensed AV delay
This is the time interval between a sensed atrial event, and the delivery of a paced ventricular stimulus. The sensed AV delay (Figure 1.14b) will therefore only be applicable to a pacemaker that is programmed in a mode including sensing in the atrium, pacing in the ventricle, and a triggered response. Examples of such settings might be DDD or VAT.

AV delay and intrinsic AV conduction
If intrinsic conduction is more rapid than the duration of the programmed AV delay (Figure 1.14c and d), the intrinsic QRS will inhibit ventricular pacing, so long as the pacing mode includes ventricular sensing.

Upper rate limit

There are two types of upper rate limit: upper sensor rate, and upper tracking rate. To have an upper sensor rate, the rate-response sensor must be programmed "on" (see section on "Basic pacemaker programming – sensing, pacing, and refractory periods"). In other words, the mode (see section on "Pacing modes") must be rate responsive (e.g. VVIR or DDDR). To have an upper tracking rate, the device must be in a triggered or tracking mode (see sections on "Conceptual building blocks of pacemaker function and Pacing modes").

Upper sensor rate limit

A single or dual chamber pacemaker in a rate-response mode (see section on "Basic pacemaker programming – sensing, pacing, and refractory periods") will have an upper sensor rate. This is the maximum rate at which the sensor will drive the pacemaker. For example, if the sensor upper rate is set at 120 bpm, then the pacemaker will pace at 120 bpm when the sensor is maximally activated (unless the patient's heart rate is even higher and inhibits pacing).

Upper tracking rate

In a dual chamber pacemaker programmed to a *triggered mode* (e.g. DDD or VAT), the upper tracking rate is the maximum atrial rate at which a pacemaker will deliver a ventricular pacing stimulus following each sensed atrial beat (i.e. in a 1 : 1 ratio). For example, if the upper tracking rate is set at 120 bpm, and the atrial rate is 130 bpm, the pacemaker will not deliver a ventricular pacing stimulus after each P wave. If it did, then it would be pacing the ventricle also at 130 bpm, and this would be said to "violate" the upper rate limit. If programmed correctly, the pacemaker rate will plateau at about 120 bpm. If the atrial rate is 130 bpm, and the ventricular rate is 120 bpm, this will have an appearance somewhat like Wenckebach conduction (see Figure 1.15). This, therefore, is sometimes referred to as pseudo-Wenckebach or pacemaker-Wenckebach behavior. The programming issues surrounding upper rate behavior are discussed below.

Upper rate behavior

Upper rate behavior describes the response of a dual chamber pacemaker, programmed in a tracking mode, to increasing atrial rates. The upper rate behaviors described below will be most apparent in patients who are dependent on the pacemaker for AV conduction. In patients with intact AV conduction, *competition* from intrinsic conduction (see section on "Competition and fusion") may partially mask these behaviors. An example of a situation in which the upper rate response of a pacemaker would be important would be a patient with complete heart block, who has a dual chamber pacemaker programmed in DDD mode, and is exercising. Upper rate behavior combines the concepts of AV delay, upper tracking rate (discussed in the section on

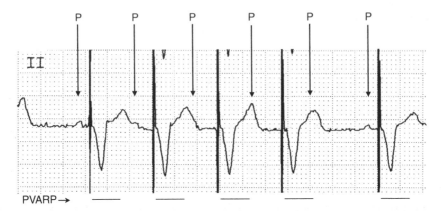

Figure 1.15 Upper rate behavior of a properly programmed pacemaker. The sinus rate is 120 bpm, and the pacemaker upper tracking rate is 110 bpm. The arrows indicate P waves. The heavy vertical black lines are ventricular pacing stimuli. The horizontal black bars below the tracing indicate the duration of the PVARP after each pacing stimulus. The pacemaker delays the ventricular stimulus (increases the AV delay) progressively after each P wave, so that the upper rate limit is not violated. When the penultimate P wave falls into the PVARP, it is not tracked and the cycle begins again.

"Basic pacemaker programming – timing cycles"), and PVARP (see section on "Basic pacemaker programming – sensing, pacing, and refractory periods"). If the atrial rate becomes fast enough, the pacemaker will stop tracking every atrial beat. Depending on the atrial rate, and pacemaker programming, the ECG may have the appearance of Wenckebach AV block (sometimes called pacemaker Wenckebach or pseudo-Wenckebach) or sudden 2 : 1 AV block. Under some circumstances, the pacemaker may stop tracking all atrial beats (mode switch).

Wenckebach upper rate response
When the atrial rate just exceeds the upper tracking rate, the pacemaker prolongs the AV delay progressively so that the ventricular pacing stimuli are not delivered at a rate faster than the upper rate limit (Figure 1.15). Therefore, as the AV delay gets progressively longer, the P wave gets closer to the preceding paced ventricular beat, until eventually the P wave is within the PVARP of the preceding beat, and that P wave is not tracked. This is the way that a properly programmed dual chamber pacemaker will behave when the atrial rate increases to, and is then above, the programmed upper tracking rate.

2 : 1 upper rate response
Sometimes, a pacemaker is improperly programmed such that the P wave encroaches on the preceding PVARP at an atrial rate at or below the upper rate limit of the pacemaker. In this case, the AV delay will not prolong. Instead, the pacemaker will suddenly track 2 : 1. That is, it will deliver one

(a)

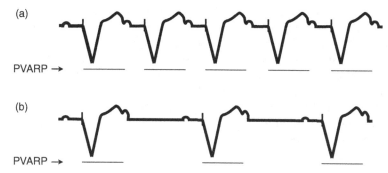

PVARP →

(b)

PVARP →

Figure 1.16 Upper rate behavior of an improperly programmed pacemaker. This patient does not have intrinsic AV conduction. The sinus rate is similar to Figure 1.15. The horizontal black bars below the tracings indicate the duration of the PVARP. Note that both the programmed AV delay, and the PVARP are longer than in Figure 1.15. In (a), the sinus rate is just slow enough so that the P wave does not fall into the PVARP of the preceding paced ventricular beat. In (b), the sinus rate has increased slightly, such that every second P wave falls into the PVARP of the preceding paced beat. P waves falling in the PVARP are not tracked, and so ventricular pacing does not occur after these P waves. The result is a sudden change from 1 : 1 to 2 : 1 AV conduction. (If the programmed lower pacing rate is greater than the 2 : 1 block rate, then ventricular pacing will not fall below this rate.) To allow 1 : 1 tracking at the sinus rate shown in the figure, the pacemaker must be reprogrammed to a shorter PVARP or shorter sensed AV delay, or both.

ventricular pacing impulse for every two atrial impulses (Figure 1.16). For example, a pacemaker programmed in this way might suddenly change ventricular pacing rate from 120 bpm (1 : 1 AV conduction) to 61 bpm (2 : 1 AV conduction) as the patient's sinus rate increased from 120 to 122 bpm. A sudden decrease in heart rate like this during exercise would normally cause symptoms.

Proper programming of upper rate limit, sensed AV delay, and PVARP will ensure a smooth transition from 1 : 1 tracking to Wenckebach, and then to 2 : 1 tracking as the heart rate increases. The details of how to program a pacemaker for correct upper rate behavior are beyond the scope of this chapter, but can be found in the references listed in the bibliography.

Mode switching

Mode switching is, as the term suggests, an automatic change from a triggered mode (e.g. DDD) to a nontriggered mode (e.g. DDI). This feature was developed to deal with the problem of the response of a pacemaker programmed in a triggered mode to atrial tachyarrhythmias, such as atrial fibrillation. Such rapid atrial arrhythmias would otherwise cause sustained high ventricular rates in triggered modes. Ventricular tracking of a rapid atrial rate is physiological during exercise, but if the rapid atrial rate is caused by an arrhythmia, ventricular tracking at the upper rate limit is not desirable.

When a pacemaker with mode switch capability, programmed to the DDD mode, senses a very rapid atrial rate, it automatically switches to a nontracking mode. (The patient may still have rapid intrinsic conduction, and a rapid ventricular response, but it will not be due to the pacemaker.) In practice, the pacemaker uses an atrial rate threshold to distinguish sinus tachycardia from atrial arrhythmias such as atrial flutter, which can have an atrial rate of 300 bpm, or atrial fibrillation, which is even faster. When the atrial rate falls below the rate programmed for mode switch, then the pacemaker changes back to a tracking mode.

Competition and fusion

Competition describes the relationship between intrinsic beats and paced beats in a chamber, when both are present. If the surface QRS morphology is a blend of the intrinsic QRS and the paced QRS, it is said to be *fused*. There can be competition between an intrinsic pacemaker (such as the sinus node) and an implanted pacemaker (Figure 1.17). There can also be competition between intrinsic AV conduction and dual chamber pacing of the ventricle (Figure 1.18). If intrinsic AV conduction is intact, then ventricular pacing that follows a sensed or paced atrial beat may *compete* with intrinsic QRS complexes resulting from intact AV conduction. In other words, there will be a race to capture the ventricle. If the electrical activity resulting from the paced beat spreads throughout the heart before intrinsic conduction progresses through the His-Purkinje system, then the QRS complex is broad, and is said to be *fully paced*.

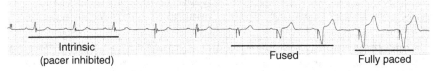

Intrinsic
(pacer inhibited)   Fused   Fully paced

Figure 1.17 VVI pacing competing with sinus rhythm. This illustrates fusion, as well the concepts of inhibition and competition. The pacemaker is programmed in VVI mode at a rate of 60 bpm. The patient's sinus rate is initially 61 bpm at the beginning of the strip, but then slows slightly to about 58 bpm by the end of the strip. Thus the sinus node *competes* with the pacemaker for control of the heart rhythm. At the beginning of the strip, the pacemaker is *inhibited* by sinus rhythm (no pacemaker stimuli are seen), and so the *intrinsic* QRS morphology is seen. At the end of the strip, the ventricle is fully paced, and a paced QRS morphology is seen. (Note that the P wave is not affected, as this pacemaker is not programmed to pace or sense in the atrium.) In the middle of the strip, the QRS morphology is a combination of the intrinsic QRS seen on the left of the strip, and the paced QRS seen on the right of the strip. It is therefore said to be *fused*. (The fourth and fifth complexes on the strip show a pacer stimulus artifact in front of a fully intrinsic QRS. This is called pseudofusion.)

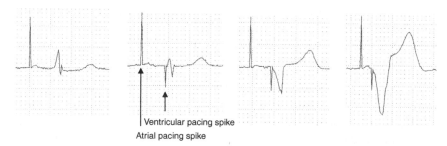

Ventricular pacing spike

Atrial pacing spike

Figure 1.18 Competition between DDD pacing and intrinsic AV conduction. The large amplitude signal before each P wave is the atrial pacing stimulus artifact. The pacemaker is set in DDD mode. The AV delay is programmed to progressively shorter values in each panel from left to right. [(a) 300 ms, (b) 220 ms, (c) 190 ms, and (d) 100 ms.] (a) shows intrinsic AV conduction following a paced atrial complex. Ventricular pacing is inhibited by the intrinsic QRS complex, which therefore must have been sensed by the ventricular channel of the pacemaker prior to the end of the programmed AV delay. (b) and (c) show fusion of ventricular pacing and intrinsic conduction. (d) shows a fully paced QRS complex.

Frequently asked questions: interpretation of pacing behavior on telemetry and ECGs (questions that arise from normal pacemaker behavior)

Arrhythmia services frequently field questions regarding pacing behavior seen on telemetry monitors and on ECGs. As a general rule, if the pacemaker or defibrillator was implanted more than a few weeks ago, and is followed on a regular basis, malfunction is quite rare. The vast majority of questions we receive are the result of normal pacemaker behavior. The following section includes frequently asked questions grouped by the type of pacemaker behavior, and a description of normal pacemaker behavior that may account for them.

"I don't see pacemaker spikes"

1 The pacemaker may not be pacing: this is usually due to inhibition by the patient's intrinsic heart rate, which may be faster than the lower rate limit of the pacemaker.
2 The pacemaker may be pacing, but the stimulus artifacts (spikes) are not visible: unipolar pacing stimulus artifacts are large and nearly always visible. Bipolar pacing stimulus artifacts, however, may be too small in amplitude to see. In addition, certain monitors do not have sufficiently rapid frequency response to detect pacemaker stimuli in their usual recording mode, and must specifically be set to detect pacing.

"The pacer is pacing too slowly"

1 Inaccurate heart rate reading from the cardiac monitor: a cardiac monitor's numerical display of heart rate may be inaccurate. The correct way

to determine heart rate is to print an ECG strip and measure the heart rate manually.

2 Hysteresis: hysteresis is the term for a pacemaker function that allows heart rates to go below the lower rate limit of the pacemaker. If the pacemaker is set to a lower rate limit of 60 bpm, with a hysteresis of 50 bpm, then the pacemaker will allow the intrinsic heart rate to drop until it reaches 50. At this point, the pacemaker will begin pacing at the lower rate limit of 60. It will continue to pace at that rate until the patient's intrinsic heart rate becomes faster than the pacemaker's lower rate limit. Once the intrinsic heart rate takes over from the pacer, then the intrinsic heart rate may again drop from above 60 bpm down to 50 bpm before pacing again occurs.

3 Sleep function: some pacemakers can be set for a reduced pacing rate during the time period when the patient would be expected to be asleep, so that the patient is not bothered by pacing that is more rapid than is physiologically necessary during sleep.

"The heart rate is going too fast"

1 Intrinsic rhythm: it is important to remember that pacemakers treat only slow heart rhythms. Pacemakers (with rare exceptions) cannot slow a rapid rhythm. (Defibrillators may treat certain types of rapid heart rhythms; this will be presented in a later chapter.) To distinguish between pacing and intrinsic rhythm, look for pacing stimulus artifacts before the atrial or QRS complexes. If these are not visible, and if the QRS complexes are narrow, then the rhythm is probably intrinsic. A rapid and markedly irregular rhythm usually suggests atrial fibrillation.

2 Tracking of atrial rapid rhythm: a pacemaker set to DDD, or another triggered mode, will track a rapid atrial rhythm. Each atrial beat will be followed by a ventricular paced beat (unless inhibited by more rapid intrinsic conduction) up to the *upper tracking rate*. The upper tracking rate can be programmed: 120 bpm is a common default setting, but it can range up to 180 bpm. The pacemaker will not pace the ventricle any faster than the upper rate limit is set (see discussion of upper rate limits above). Ventricular tracking of sinus or atrial tachycardia is a common source of confusion. In order assess this behavior, look carefully at the 12-lead ECG to see if there are intrinsic P waves before every paced ventricular beat. If so, the rapid ventricular pacing is due to tracking of a rapid atrial rate (see Figure 1.9 above). The treatment for this (if needed) is directed toward the cause of the rapid intrinsic atrial rate.

3 Rate response: as noted above, current pacemakers and defibrillators can be set to be rate responsive. Increased minute ventilation or motion of the device can sometimes inappropriately activate the sensors. Examples might be hyperventilation, physical therapy, manipulation of the shoulder area. To make this diagnosis, examine a 12-lead ECG. If the pacemaker is in DDD mode, there will be dual chamber (AV sequential) pacing. If there is atrial pacing before every ventricular paced beat, then this diagnosis is in play.

If the atrial activity is intrinsic, then it is simply ventricular tracking of a rapid atrial rhythm (see item 2 above). If the pacemaker is a single chamber ventricular pacer, then atrial activity will not bear a constant relationship to the paced ventricular activity. If the device is a single chamber atrial pacer, then of course, only the atrium will be paced, with intrinsic conduction to the ventricle.

4 Rate smoothing algorithm: some pacemakers and defibrillators can be set to smooth out heart rate variations. This feature prevents abrupt slowing of the heart rate, which may be responsible for certain arrhythmias. Premature beats, such as a run of premature atrial complexes (PACs) or PVCs, may be followed by pacing above the lower rate limit. The pacing rate will then gradually slow down, unless there are more premature beats.

5 PMT: this is discussed in the section on "Basic pacemaker programming – sensing, pacing, and refractory periods" under the heading "Refractory period," and in Figure 1.13.

"Pacemaker spikes are where they shouldn't be"

1 Monitor artifact: monitors that do not have sufficiently fast frequency response to actually record pacemaker stimuli may attempt to mark pacemaker depolarization by using a vertical black line (i.e. these monitors create a stimulus artifact). If the marking is incorrect, then these lines may appear in places where pacemaker depolarization is not actually present.

2 Ventricular sensing which occurs late in the QRS: as noted above (see section on "Conceptual building blocks of pacemaker function"), it is not the onset of the QRS complex that inhibits the ventricular channel output, but the actual arrival of the sensed R wave signal at the ventricular channel of the pacemaker via the ventricular lead. This is likely to happen after the onset of the QRS complex, and the pacemaker can deliver a ventricular pacing stimulus before it is "aware" that there is a QRS complex in progress.

3 Crosschannel blanking and safety pacing: this is a common source of pacing stimulus artifacts occurring in the ST segment (Figure 1.19).

"What is it?"

If a ventricular sensed beat occurs at the same time as an atrial paced beat, the pacemaker will deliver a ventricular pacing stimulus. This feature is usually activated when a PVC occurs at exactly the time that the atrial pacing stimulus is delivered, so that the pacemaker senses a beat in the ventricular chamber at the same time that it is delivering an atrial pacing stimulus. The pacemaker will then deliver a ventricular stimulus, even though it just sensed a ventricular event, resulting in a pacemaker stimulus later in the QRS complex or in the ST segment of the PVC (Figure 1.19). This is frequently mistaken for pacemaker malfunction. The way to determine if normal pacemaker behavior is occurring, is to march out the atrial stimulus artifacts using calipers. If there is an early ventricular depolarization (a PVC), which falls at the same time as the atrial stimulus, and there is a ventricular stimulus in the ST segment, or T wave, this is normal pacemaker behavior.

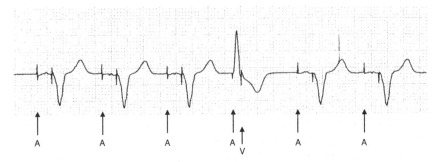

Figure 1.19 Crosschannel blanking/safety pacing behavior. Atrial pacing stimulus artifacts are labeled "A". A PVC happens to occur simultaneously with the fourth atrial pacing stimulus. The pacemaker thus has sensed an event on the ventricular channel, occurring nearly simultaneously with the pacing output on the atrial channel. The concern is that the sensed event on the ventricular channel might actually be the atrial pacing stimulus, rather than an intrinsic QRS. (The pacemaker cannot tell the difference; they both would be simply an electrical signal.) To make sure that a ventricular beat occurs, the pacemaker delivers a ventricular pacing stimulus V. If there is already an intrinsic QRS complex, the pacing will do no harm, but if the ventricular channel is instead sensing the atrial pacing stimulus, a ventricular paced beat may prevent asystole. The difference between this AV delay and the normal paced AV delay depends on the manufacturer. To recognize this, march out the atrial stimulus artifacts. If one coincides with a PVC, and is followed by another stimulus artifact, consider this type of behavior.

"Why do pacemakers have this feature?"
An understanding of the reason for the feature may aid in recognizing it. In dual chamber pacemakers, there is the concern that atrial pacing might be sensed by the ventricular lead. This might occur if the atrial pacing output is large in amplitude, is close to the ventricle, or if the atrial pacing lead dislodges and falls into the ventricle, and paces without capturing the ventricle. If the ventricular channel is inhibited by the atrial pacing stimulus which the pacemaker interprets as a QRS complex, then asystole may result if there is no intrinsic ventricular rhythm.

Differential diagnosis: failure of the pacemaker to sense in the ventricle, or oversensing in the atrium followed by triggered ventricular activity, can be a cause of similar behavior. These subjects are beyond the scope of this chapter. If there is any question about the behavior, the strip should be reviewed with a pacemaker specialist.

References

1 Barold SS, Stroobandt R, Sinnaeve F. *Cardiac pacemakers step by step: an illustrated guide.* Oxford: Blackwell Futura Publishing Co., 2004.
2 Hesselson A. *Simplified interpretations of pacemaker ECGs.* Oxford: Blackwell Publishing, 2003.

3 Ellenbogen K, Wood M. *Cardiac pacing and ICDs*. Oxford: Blackwell Publishing, 2005.
4 Hayes DL, Lloyd MA, Friedman PA. *Cardiac pacing and defibrillation: a clinical approach.* New York: Futura Publishing Co., 2000.
5 Ellenbogen K, Kay GN, Wilkoff BL. *Clinical cardiac pacing and defibrillation*. Philadelphia: W.B. Saunders, 2000.
6 Love CJ. *Handbook of cardiac pacing*. Georgetown, Texas: Landes Bioscience, 1998.
7 Hayes DL *Cardiac pacemakers and implantable defibrillators: a workbook in 3 volumes. Volume 1: Cardiac pacing: a case approach*. New York: Futura Publishing Co., 1998.
8 Christiansen J. *Cardiac pacemakers and implantable defibrillators: a workbook in 3 volumes. Volume 3: Transtelephonic electrocardiography and troubelshooting: a case approach*. New York: Futura Publishing Co., 1998.
9 Sutton R, Stack Z, Heaven D *et al.* Mode switching for atrial tachyarrhythmias. *Am J Cardiol* 1999; 83: 11.
10 Hayes DL, Vlietstra RE. Pacemaker malfunction. *Ann Inter Med* 1993; 119: 828–35.
11 Garson A, Jr. Stepwise approach to the unknown pacemaker ECG. *Am Heart J* 1990; 119: 924–41.

Glossary

Asynchronous: Pacing that is not inhibited by intrinsic beats (see Figure 1.11).

Bipolar pacing: Pacing stimulus delivery between the tip and the ring electrodes of a bipolar pacing lead.

Bipolar sensing: Sensing of intrinsic electrical activity between the tip and the ring electrodes of a bipolar pacing lead.

Capture: The actual excitation or depolarization of cardiac tissue by a pacing stimulus. A pacing stimulus might be too weak to actually depolarize surrounding cardiac tissue, or the tissue might be refractory, in which case the pacing stimulus is said to *fail to capture*.

Channel: The lead input and circuitry on a pacemaker dedicated to a particular chamber of the heart. For example, in a dual chamber pacemaker, the ventricular channel receives sensed beats from the ventricular lead, and transmits the ventricular pacing impulse to the ventricular lead.

Compete: What two independent sources of depolarization may do (see Figures 1.17 and 1.18).

Depolarized: The initial state of activation of cardiac tissue.

Excitable: Cardiac tissue is said to be *excitable* when it can be activated by a pacing stimulus or an intrinsic wave of depolarization. The opposite of this is *refractory*.

Fully paced: A beat or series of beats that result (at least as far as is visible on the surface ECG) only from pacing, in contrast to *fused* beats or *intrinsically conducted* beats.

Fused: The QRS appearance of beats that result from a combination of activation via a pacing stimulus, and intrinsic activation, occurring simultaneously.

Heart block: The absence of intrinsic conduction between the atria and the ventricles.

*Intrinsic beat (*also *intrinsic depolarization, intrinsic complex)*: A P wave or QRS complex arising from the heart's own electrical activity, in contrast to a *paced beat*.

Intrinsic conduction: Conduction of an atrial impulse (sensed or paced) via the His-Purkinje system, causing an intrinsic ventricular QRS complex. Intrinsic conduction may be absent, in which case there is heart block, or masked by ventricular paced beats occurring before the intrinsic impulse has had a chance to make its way through the His-Purkinje system to activate the ventricle.

Lead: The insulated wire that runs from the pacemaker or defibrillator pulse generator into the heart.

Mode: A description of the general way a pacemaker is programmed to pace. This is described by a code of letters, which specifies which chambers are paced, and in what ways. See Chapter 3 for a more complete description.

Oversensing: Sensing on a channel of a pacemaker of something other than what that channel is supposed to sense. For example, if the ventricular channel of a pacemaker sensed the T wave, an atrial pacing stimulus, or electrical noise from a lead fracture (and therefore the pacemaker interpreted one of these signals as QRS complexes) the ventricular channel would be *oversensing*.

P wave: Atrial activity, on the surface ECG, or as sensed by the pacemaker or defibrillator.

Paced AV delay: The delay between the delivery of the atrial pacing stimulus and the delivery of the ventricular pacing stimulus.

*Paced beat (*also *paced complex)*: A P wave or QRS complex initiated by pacing, in contrast to an *intrinsic beat*.

Postventricular atrial refractory period (PVARP): The period after a ventricular sensed or paced event, when the atrial channel is refractory.

Polarized: The state of the cardiac cell membrane prior to activation (*depolarization*). This refers to the separation of positive and negative charges on the outside and inside of the cell, respectively.

Programmable: A pacemaker parameter that can be altered by using the manufacturer's programmer is said to be programmable.

Programmer: A portable device that allows communication with the pacemaker or defibrillator via an electromagnetic telemetry link. This link allows downloading of stored information from the pacemaker or defibrillator, and programming of various parameters. Programmers are specific to the pacemaker brand.

Pulse generator: The main body of the pacemaker or defibrillator that houses the battery and circuits.

R wave: The intrinsic QRS complex, as sensed by the pacemaker or defibrillator.

Refractory: Cardiac tissue is said to be *refractory* when it cannot be activated by a pacing stimulus or an intrinsic wave of depolarization. The opposite of this is *excitable*.

Refractory period: When the term is applied to cardiac tissue, this is the period of time after a depolarization during which the tissue cannot be electrically excited. The exact definition is the time between an electrical stimulus that excites a certain part of the heart, and the latest subsequent stimulus that cannot excite the same tissue. When the term is applied to a pacemaker, it refers to the period after a sensed or paced beat during which the pacemaker will ignore another sensed event. This is a programmable parameter.

Retrograde: Electrical activity moving in the direction opposite to normal (which is anterograde).

Sensed AV delay: The time interval between a sensed atrial event, and the delivery of a paced ventricular stimulus.

Sensed beat: An intrinsic R wave or P wave that has been registered by the pacemaker or defibrillator. Similar to *intrinsic beat*, but with the added requirement that the pacemaker has actually sensed (or registered) the beat.

Sensing: The function of detecting the intrinsic electrical activity of the heart.

Sensitivity: A description of the level of the sensing function. The setting of this function gives the minimum amplitude of intrinsic electrical activity that the pacemaker will register. For example, if the sensitivity in the ventricular chamber of the pacemaker is set to 5 mV, the intrinsic R wave must transmit an electrical signal at least 5 mV in amplitude for the pacemaker to register that an intrinsic beat has occurred.

Settings: The way a pacemaker is programmed.

Stimulus: The electrical output delivered by a pacemaker, through a pacemaker lead to the heart, in order to pace the heart.

Stimulus artifact: The mark created by a pacemaker stimulus on the surface ECG or telemetry monitor.

Tracking: A normal behavior of dual chamber pacing in a triggered mode. The pacemaker senses activity in one chamber (usually the atrium) and delivers a pacing *stimulus* in the other chamber (usually the ventricle) after a certain time delay (the AV delay).

Triggered mode: A pacing mode in which a sensed beat triggers a paced beat. This is most commonly used in a dual chamber pacemaker, so that a sensed atrial beat triggers a paced ventricular beat, after an adjustable delay. In this setting, the ventricle is said to be *tracking* the atrium.

Unipolar pacing: Pacing stimulus delivery between the electrode of pacing lead and the shell of the pulse generator.

Unipolar sensing: Sensing of intrinsic electrical activity between the electrode of pacing lead and the shell of the pulse generator.

Wenckebach upper rate response (also known as *pseudo-Wenckebach*, and *pacemaker Wenckebach*): A progressive increase in the interval between an intrinsic atrial beat and the ventricular pacing stimulus, culminating in an atrial beat that is not followed by ventricular pacing, after which the cycle begins again (Figure 1.15). This occurs in dual chamber pacemakers, programmed in a tracking mode, at atrial rates just above the upper tracking rate limit (see section on "Upper rate behavior").

CHAPTER 2

Temporary cardiac pacing

Oliver R. Segal, Vias Markides, D. Wyn Davies, and Nicholas S. Peters

Background

Following its inception in the 1950s, temporary cardiac pacing has revolutionized the emergency treatment of profound bradyarrhythmias. It offers the ability to artificially increase atrial and/or ventricular heart rates until such time as the precipitant of the bradycardia disappears or is corrected, or permanent pacing can be performed. Several different approaches to temporary cardiac pacing exist but all rely on an external pulse generator to supply sufficient current via easily removable electrodes to initiate cardiac contraction. It was first developed using electrodes attached via hypodermic needles through the chest wall by Paul Zoll in 1952 for the treatment of ventricular standstill.[1] By 1958 Furman and Robinson had described the first transvenous endocardial pacing approach.[2,3] Currently, external (transcutaneous), endocardial, epicardial and transesophageal/gastric approaches exist for temporary cardiac pacing all of which enable rapid correction of circulatory integrity in patients presenting with inadequate heart rates.

In addition to the management of bradycardia, temporary pacing technology has been adapted for use in the emergency treatment of tachyarrhythmias. Initially described by Waldo *et al.* for the treatment of atrial flutter following open heart surgery, continuous rapid pacing was performed via temporarily implanted epicardial atrial electrodes to induce 2 : 1 atrioventricular (AV) block, thereby reducing the ventricular rate.[4] This technique, called overdrive pacing, has subsequently been refined so that many supraventricular[5] and ventricular tachycardias[6] can be terminated using transvenous pacing wires in the emergency setting, thereby avoiding the need for external cardioversion. It is even possible to terminate these arrhythmias using external[7] and transesophageal pacing approaches.[8]

Indications

The indications for temporary cardiac pacing can be divided into the emergency treatment of bradyarrhythmias [most commonly complicating myocardial infarction (MI)], tachyarrhythmias, and prophylactic pacing for the at-risk patient prior to surgery or other procedure. Indications are summarised in Table 2.1.

Table 2.1 Indications for temporary pacing

Bradyarrhythmias associated with MI
 1 Asystole
 2 Complete AV block
 3 Second-degree AV block
 4 Bradycardia-dependent ventricular arrhythmias
 5 Sinus bradycardia
 6 RBBB and LBBB
 7 Bifascicular block with first-degree AV block

Bradyarrhythmias not associated with MI
 1 Asystole
 2 Complete AV block
 3 Second-degree AV block
 4 Bradycardia-dependent ventricular arrhythmias
 5 Drug overdose (e.g. β blockers, digoxin, verapamil)

Bradyarrhythmias requiring temporary dual chamber pacing
 1 Bradyarrhythmias listed above–when associated with acute severe circulatory failure, cardiogenic shock, and pulmonary edema, especially when ventricular pacing alone fails to improve circulatory function

*Tachyarrhythmias**
 1 Atrial tachycardia
 2 Atrial flutter
 3 AVNRT
 4 AVRT
 5 VT (sustained, monomorphic)
 6 Torsades de pointes

Prophylactic temporary pacing for surgery/procedures

Bradyarrhythmias requiring temporary pacing in patients undergoing GA
 1 Second- or third-degree AV block
 2 Bifascicular block and first-degree AV block[†]
 3 LBBB and first-degree AV block[†]

Procedures which may induce bradycardia
 1 Elective replacement of permanent pacemaker generator
 2 Cardiac surgery
 3 Neurosurgical procedures
 4 Thoracic sympathectomy
 5 Carotid surgery
 6 Right coronary angioplasty

GA=general anesthesia
*Overdrive pacing via a temporary pacing wire is indicated for sustained, drug-refractory arrhythmias, especially if hemodynamically unstable.
[†]No clear benefit has been demonstrated for prophylactic temporary pacing in patients with bifascicular block and first-degree AV block, and for those with LBBB and first-degree AV block in patients requiring GA. See text for details.

Bradyarrhythmias

The primary complications of profound bradyarrhythmias that are reversible with temporary pacing are failure of circulatory function [hypotension, syncope, asystole, cardiogenic shock and failure of cerebral function (confusion and coma)] and bradycardia-related ventricular arrhythmias. The most common setting in which these complications occur is acute MI; temporary cardiac pacing is indicated when any of these complications arise. The bradyarrhythmias for which temporary cardiac pacing is indicated are outlined below, which is based upon the American College of Cardiology/American Heart Association Guidelines for the management of patients with acute MI published in 1999.[9]

Bradyarrhythmias associated with MI

Importantly, thrombolytic treatment or percutaneous coronary intervention should not be delayed by the need for temporary pacing, although the two may need to be instituted concurrently.

Asystole
Patients presenting with episodes of asystole should be treated with temporary cardiac pacing.

Complete AV block
Complete AV block is seen in ~5% of patients presenting with acute MI and is usually seen within the first 48 h after the onset of symptoms.[10] The arterial blood supply to the AV node arises from the right coronary artery in ~80% of the patients and from the circumflex artery in the remainder,[11] and is therefore most frequently seen with infarction of the inferior wall. Complete heart block is also seen in anterior MI due to widespread ischemic damage to the basal septal structures including the bundle of His, usually due to occlusion of the left anterior descending artery prior to the first septal perforator branch. Therefore, complete heart block, which complicates anterior MI, is associated with extensive myocardial necrosis as well as worse prognosis.

The degree of bradycardia associated with complete AV block is dependent on the site of the block and, subsequently, the origin of the ventricular escape rhythm. Junctional escape rhythms (originating from close to the bundle of His and usually associated with inferior MI) are seen when the site of block is close to, or at, the level of the AV node. Typically, electrocardiogram (ECG) complexes have a normal or nearly normal QRS width and heart rates often compatible with normal circulatory function (Figure 2.1). Escape rhythms originating from infranodal structures (the bundle branches, Purkinje fibers, or ventricular muscle), and therefore usually associated with anterior MI, are frequently slower with a broad QRS (Figure 2.2). These are unreliable (and sometimes absent altogether) and may cause circulatory failure, impairment of consciousness, or sudden death; therefore emergency temporary pacing is indicated. In the majority of patients, resolution of AV block occurs following

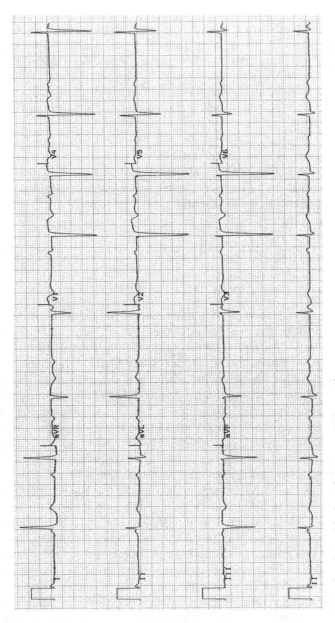

Figure 2.1 Complete heart block with narrow QRS complex escape.

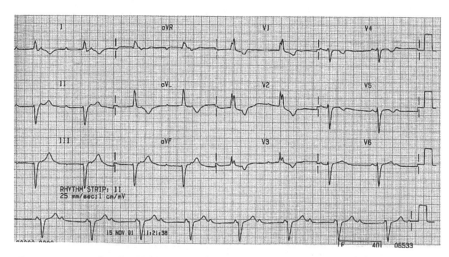

Figure 2.2 Complete heart block with broad QRS complex escape (right bundle branch block).

thrombolytic therapy or revascularization, however, a proportion of patients will require permanent pacing because of persistent AV block.

Second-degree AV block
Second degree AV block is also frequently seen following MI. Möbitz Type II AV block (intermittent AV block with no change in PR interval during AV conduction, Figure 2.3) is almost always infranodal and if the associated brady-cardia results in hemodynamic compromise or neurological symptoms, then temporary pacing is indicated. Möbitz Type I AV block (Wenckebach block: visible, differing, and generally decremental PR intervals) when associated with a narrow QRS complex (Figure 2.4a) is almost always AV nodal, but if associated with bundle branch block (Figure 2.4b) is commonly associated with infranodal block.[12] Möbitz Type I AV block infrequently leads to impair-ment of circulatory function but if symptomatic, despite atropine, will require pacing. Importantly, ~20% of patients presenting with Möbitz Type I block in the setting of acute MI will progress to Möbitz Type II or complete heart block and therefore, close monitoring is required.[13]

Sinus bradycardia
Sinus bradycardia (rate <50/min) in the context of MI should initially be treated with atropine and/or isoprenaline. However, if the patient remains symptomatic and systolic blood pressure is <80 mm Hg, temporary cardiac pacing is indicated.

Right and left bundle branch block
Right bundle branch block (RBBB) and left bundle branch block (LBBB) can clearly not exist simultaneously without causing asystole. In isolation, neither

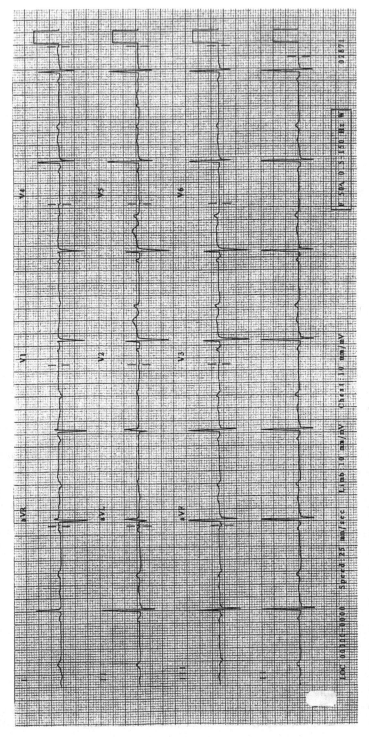

Figure 2.3 Möbitz Type II AV block (all or no conduction).

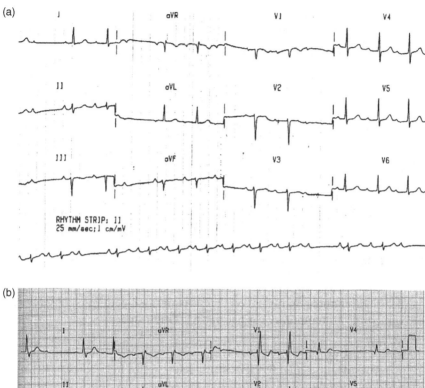

Figure 2.4 (a) Möbitz Type I AV block or Wenckebach block associated with a narrow QRS complex. (b) Möbitz Type I AV block or Wenckebach block associated with a broad QRS complex (RBBB).

of these are indications for temporary pacing and both are frequently seen during acute MI. However, alternating RBBB and LBBB can occur and has a high rate of progression to complete AV block. Similarly, the presence of RBBB and alternating left anterior hemiblock and left posterior hemiblock (i.e. alternating block in the left anterior and posterior fascicles, respectively) often predates complete AV block and both conditions imply block at the His

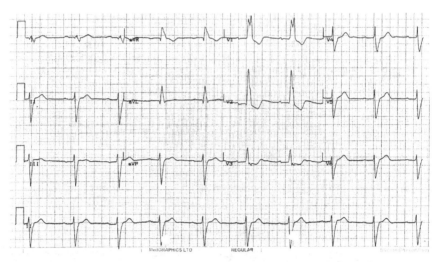

Figure 2.5 Bifascicular block (RBBB + left anterior hemiblock) and first-degree AV block.

bundle or both bundle branches. When either of these patterns is observed in the context of MI, temporary cardiac pacing is indicated.

Bifascicular block with first-degree AV block
The presence of bifascicular block (RBBB + left anterior hemiblock or RBBB + left posterior hemiblock or LBBB) and first-degree AV block (PR interval >200 ms) in the context of acute MI is an indication for temporary cardiac pacing (Figure 2.5). In the setting of acute MI this should be performed regardless of whether this block pattern is new or of indeterminate age. However, solitary bundle branch block or fascicular block that are known to exist prior to MI is not an indication for temporary cardiac pacing.

Bradyarrhythmias not associated with MI
Bradyarrhythmias in the absence of MI present less frequently with acute circulatory or cerebral impairment. However, temporary cardiac pacing is indicated (1) for patients presenting with asystole, second-degree or complete heart block with associated compromise; if permanent pacing cannot be provided immediately or if a likely transient reversible cause is identified; or (2) for bradycardia-dependent ventricular arrhythmias. Temporary cardiac pacing is also indicated in drug-induced symptomatic bradycardia, most notably from β blockers, digoxin, or verapamil.

Bradyarrhythmias requiring dual chamber temporary pacing
Dual chamber pacing, that is, pacing both right atrium and ventricle, requires the placement of two endocardial wires. Pacing the atrium and ventricle synchronously has been shown to improve cardiac output compared with

ventricular pacing alone, both in the settings of permanent[14–17] and temporary pacing.[18] Dual chamber pacing is therefore indicated in patients with the bradycardias listed above when associated with acute severe circulatory failure, cardiogenic shock, and pulmonary edema especially if ventricular pacing alone fails to improve circulatory function.

In addition, atrial pacing in patients with sinus node disease may also help prevent episodes of atrial fibrillation (AF), which are often poorly tolerated in those with concomitant heart failure.[19,20]

Tachyarrhythmias

Many tachyarrhythmias can be successfully and repeatedly terminated using a pacing technique known as overdrive suppression (described in detail below). This technique is indicated for patients with sustained drug-refractory arrhythmias, especially if hemodynamically unstable as a bridge to more substantive treatment. Tachycardias amenable to this technique include atrial tachycardia, atrial flutter, atrioventricular nodal reentrant tachycardia (AVNRT), accessory pathway mediated atrioventricular reciprocating tachycardia (AVRT), and monomorphic ventricular tachycardia (VT). Atrial and ventricular fibrillation (VF) and polymorphic VT cannot typically be terminated using this technique but may be prevented by temporary pacing if secondary to bradycardia.

Prophylactic pacing for surgical or other procedures

Temporary cardiac pacing can be performed electively for patients at risk of bradycardia before a planned procedure. Bradycardia and heart block may be caused by the administration of general anesthesia (GA) in patients with conduction system disease or by the effects of the procedure itself in patients with normal cardiac conduction.

Temporary pacing is indicated in patients with second- or third-degree AV block undergoing GA. Patients with bifascicular block and first-degree AV block, and first-degree AV block and LBBB can progress to complete heart block under the effects of GA;[21] therefore temporary pacing has historically been indicated. However, the available evidence suggests that this complication is rare and that sinus bradycardia and asystole are seen more frequently in these patients, which typically respond to atropine.[22–26] The benefit for prophylactic pacing in these patients therefore remains unclear.

Alternatively, temporary pacing may be required when the procedure itself induces bradycardia. The most striking example of this is during elective replacement of a pacemaker generator in patients who are pacing dependent. It is also commonly seen during or after cardiac surgery, especially with procedures involving the region of the AV node and His bundle (e.g. aortic valve replacement surgery) but may also be required during neurosurgical procedures, thoracic sympathectomy, carotid surgery, and occasionally prior to right coronary artery angioplasty.

Techniques

Transvenous temporary pacing

Temporary cardiac pacing should ideally be performed in a sterile room that allows the operator to use full aseptic technique. Good fluoroscopic imaging equipment, noninvasive hemodynamic and cardiac monitoring, and a full complement of resuscitation facilities should be available. Operators should have adequate training and should be supported by an experienced team of clinical staff.

Various routes, techniques and "tricks" exist for insertion of a transvenous temporary pacing wire, all with advantages and disadvantages. The operator should use the technique that they feel most comfortable with and which is most likely to be successful, with the least risk to the patient. However, all techniques require strict aseptic conditions and the patient should be draped extensively, as a large area around the patient is required for the wire to be manipulated. An experienced operator should be "scrubbed" and ready to assist if a junior operator is performing the procedure. A defibrillator should be available.

Vascular access

A central vein should be cannulated using the Seldinger technique with an appropriately sized pacing sheath, usually 5 or 6 French. These sheaths have a hemostatic valve allowing entry of the pacing wire without blood loss. The choice of which vein to cannulate will depend on the skills of the operator and the requirements and comfort of the patient.

The left subclavian vein should be avoided if at all possible, as this route is most frequently used for insertion of permanent pacing systems. The left internal jugular vein is not preferable either, due to the 90° bend in the left brachiocephalic vein before it drains into the superior vena cava (SVC) making lead placement difficult. Pacing from either femoral vein requires the patient to lie flat and results in the least stable wire position. Use of the femoral approach is also associated with a greater risk of infection if the wire is left in for a long duration. This route is generally reserved for prophylactic pacing prior to surgery or pacemaker generator change.

Thus, the preferred routes for patients requiring emergency pacing are the right internal jugular vein and right subclavian vein. The former allows slightly easier manipulation of the pacing wire for positioning the wire tip within the heart.

Positioning a wire at the right ventricular apex

The aim is to position the tip of the pacing wire (Figure 2.6) close to the right ventricular apex (RVA). This position offers the greatest stability but care should be taken to avoid the apex itself, which is thin walled and easily perforated.

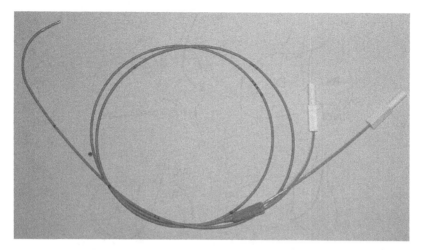

Figure 2.6 Standard 5 French transvenous pacing wire. The distal end (or pacing wire tip) has proximal and distal electrodes, and is shown on the left. The proximal end with two connectors is shown on the right.

A sterile plastic cover is included in most pacing sheath kits, which is designed to keep the proximal end of the pacing that lies outside the body sterile, although it is not used universally. If used, it should be passed over the pacing wire but left unfurled as this makes manipulating the wire significantly easier. The wire should then be advanced through the sheath into the right atrium and viewed fluoroscopically in a posteroanterior (PA) projection. The preformed curve on most pacing wires implies that the tip of the wire will curve toward the lateral wall of the right atrium (RA) (Figure 2.7a). If torque (rotation) is applied to the wire at this point, the tip will swing around so that it faces the tricuspid valve (Figure 2.7b). With the torque maintained, the wire can then be advanced through the tricuspid valve into the right ventricle toward the apex. During this point, it is normal to see ventricular ectopics stimulated by the wire touching the tricuspid valve leaflets. The wire should be rapidly moved back into the right atrium if these are continuous. If no ectopics are seen, orientation of the wire should be confirmed in a left-anterior-oblique (LAO) projection, to ensure that the wire has not been inadvertently placed in the coronary sinus or a posterior vein (Figure 2.7c).

Once in the right ventricle, the tip of the wire often remains pointing upwards toward the right ventricular outflow tract (RVOT) (Figure 2.7d). This position is not ideal as there is poor contact between the wire tip and the endocardium and stability is poor. Clockwise or anticlockwise torque should be applied and the wire simultaneously advanced or withdrawn to guide the tip toward the RVA (Figure 2.7e). Care should be taken not to apply too much torque as this may cause the whole wire to prolapse out of the ventricle and back into the right atrium. Similarly, too much pressure risks perforation. Finally, with the wire tip close to the RVA, the wire should be

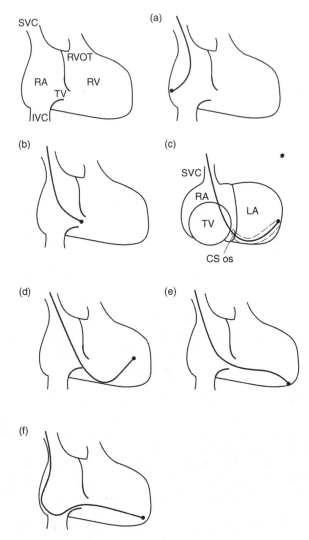

Figure 2.7 Insertion of a temporary transvenous pacing wire into the RVA.
SVC-superior vena cava, RA-right atrium, IVC-inferior vena cava, RV-right ventricle,
RVOT-right ventricular outflow tract, TV-tricuspid valve, CS os-coronary sinus os,
LA-left atrium. A diagrammatic representation of the heart is shown in a
postero-anterior projection except in panel (c) which is shown in a left
anterior-oblique (LAO) projection. Panel (a) The pacing wire is advanced into the
right atrium and the tip of the wire naturally curves towards the lateral wall. (b)
Torque is applied so that the tip faces the tricuspid valve. (c) If no ectopics are seen on
advancing the wire into the right ventricle, the wire orientation should be confirmed
in a LAO projection to ensure the wire has not been placed in the coronary sinus. (d)
Once in the right ventricle, the wire often remains pointing towards the right
ventricular outflow tract, and (e) torque should be applied whilst advancing or
withdrawing the wire to guide the tip towards the apex. (f) Once the tip is at the
apex, the wire should be carefully advanced to create a "heel" in the right atrium for
extra stability.

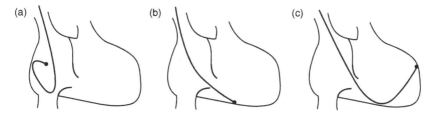

Figure 2.8 Troubleshooting techniques for transvenous temporary ventricular pacing (see text for discussion).

carefully advanced until a slight curve or "heel" is seen in the portion of the wire still in the RA (Figure 2.7f). This ensures maximum long-term stability.

Troubleshooting

The pacing wire cannot be advanced over the tricuspid valve using the technique above. The wire can be first looped within the right atrium (Figure 2.8a) and then using anticlockwise torque the wire loop can be swung around and prolapsed into the ventricle. Care should be taken when looping the wire within the right atrium, which is a thin-walled structure, to avoid forming excessive loops that may result in knotting of the wire within the atrium.

The pacing wire cannot be advanced to the RVA using the technique above. The wire should first be advanced toward the RVOT. Then, while withdrawing the wire, the tip may fall towards the apex or a small amount of torque may be required.

The pacing wire still cannot be advanced to the RVA. If the wire still cannot be advanced close to the apex, then an alternative position should be selected offering the greatest stability. A more basal portion of the inferior wall of the right ventricle can be used successfully (Figure 2.8b) and in extreme cases, the wire tip can be positioned at the RVOT for pacing if the patient has become asystolic (Figure 2.8c). This then allows the subsequent placement of another wire from a different route when the patient is more stable. However, vascular access at two different sites increases the chances of complications and the operator should be aware that manipulation of one pacing wire can dislodge another. Any position other than the RVA has relatively poor stability, especially the smooth-walled RVOT.

The pacing wire can only be advanced toward what appears to be the RVOT. Make sure that the wire is not in the coronary sinus by checking that it does not curve posteriorly in the LAO projection (Figure 2.7c).

Checking pacing parameters

Once the wire is in an anatomically suitable position close to the RVA, pacing is attempted to identify its electrical suitability. The proximal end of the pacing wire is connected to the pacing box via a connecting lead, typically using two connectors, usually with red (proximal) and black (distal) electrodes

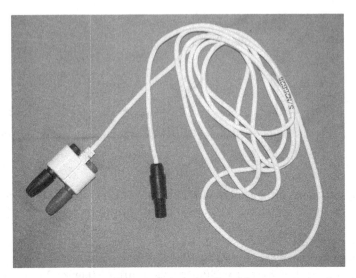

Figure 2.9 Standard connecting lead. The proximal end has two connections (red, proximal electrode and black, distal electrode) that are connected to the proximal end of the pacing wire. The distal end (center) is connected to the pacing box.

(Figure 2.9, shown in black and white). The proximal end of the connecting lead is then plugged into the pacing box; a typical example of a single lead pacing box is shown in Figure 2.10.

The pacing box has three dials to control the pacing rate, the output voltage, and the sensitivity. Before pacing is started, the pacing rate should be set at 60 beats per minute (bpm) or at least 10 bpm greater than the patient's intrinsic rate, the output voltage should be set at 3 V and the sensitivity should be set at 1 mA. The pacing box should then be switched on and capture confirmed on ECG monitoring by the presence of regular broad QRS complex beats (LBBB morphology), each preceded by a pacing spike. The ventricular rate should be the same as the rate set on the pacing box. In addition, virtually all pacing boxes will have an LED that is illuminated for each paced and each sensed beat (Figure 2.10).

If capture is demonstrated, the output voltage should be slowly reduced until loss of capture occurs. The output should then be increased until capture returns. This level is called the pacing threshold and ideally should be less than 1 V. A level up to 1.5 V is acceptable if another stable position cannot be achieved. The operator should be aware that in patients with profound bradycardia, loss of capture when reducing the output can lead to asystole. If this occurs, the output should be quickly increased until capture returns.

The stability of the wire in this position should then be checked by asking the patient to take some deep breaths, cough, and sniff while looking for episodes of loss of capture. The wire should also be viewed fluoroscopically during one

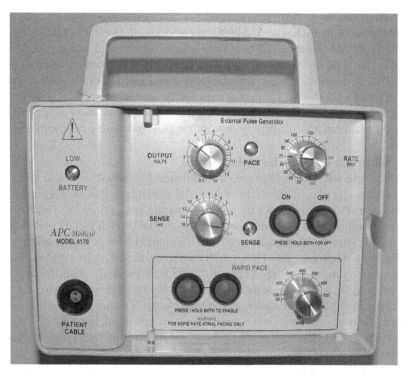

Figure 2.10 A standard single chamber temporary pacing box. The connecting lead is plugged into the socket at bottom left. The three dials at the top are for setting output voltage, pacing rate, and sensitivity. There are two LEDs in the center for displaying paced and sensed beats. The controls at the bottom are for rapid pacing.

of these maneuvers to directly examine the stability of the tip of the wire on the endocardium.

If a threshold of <1 V is obtained, the patient should usually be paced at 60–80 bpm if there is a permanent bradycardia, for example, complete heart block. If the bradycardia is intermittent, pacing at 60/min may suffice. The output voltage should be set at three times the threshold voltage and a minimum of 3 V, and the sensitivity left at 1 mA. High output voltages can lead to diaphragmatic capture, diagnosed by feeling the epigastrium moving simultaneously with pacing. When this occurs, the output voltage should be reduced, if capture can still be maintained, or if not the wire repositioned.

It is important to ensure that unless the patient's underlying rhythm is permanent asystole, the pacing mode should always have sensitivity turned on (i.e. VVI). This ensures that spontaneous ventricular depolarizations, whether normally conducted or ectopic, are sensed by the pacing box and pacing is inhibited. This prevents competitive, fixed-rate pacing (equivalent to VOO mode) in which pacing can occur during the T wave of a normally conducted beat that can lead to ventricular arrhythmias.

Securing the wire

Once the pacing wire has been adequately positioned, the sterile plastic sheath (if used) should be advanced over the wire and connected to the base of the sheath. The wire just proximal to the sheath should then be sutured into position. The rest of the wire can then be looped and secured to the patient using sutures and adhesive dressings. Care should be taken securing the wire to the patient to prevent it from being moved inadvertently. A chest X-ray should then be performed to confirm wire position and exclude a pneumothorax.

Positioning a wire in the right atrium

Atrial pacing wires typically have a preformed "J-shaped" curve at the end to enable easier placement in the right atrial appendage (RAA) (Figure 2.11), therefore these wires cannot be placed from the femoral route. The RAA is an anterior structure that has a broad base (unlike the left atrial appendage). The pacing wire should be advanced into the right atrium as with a ventricular pacing wire (Figure 2.12a). The tip of the wire should be positioned anteriorly by applying torque (Figure 2.12b) and the wire carefully withdrawn until the tip is against the endocardium and slightly opened out (Figure 2.12c). Checking the anterior positioning of the wire is made easier by screening in an oblique view on fluoroscopy. Once in the correct position, the wire tip should rock from side to side with atrial contraction; this is sometimes described as a "windscreen wiper" motion (Figure 2.12d).

Newer pacing wires are available that offer "active fixation," that is, fixation of the wire tip to the endocardium by a screw mechanism (Figure 2.13). This ensures greater lead stability over a longer period. Checking pacing parameters is the same as for a ventricular lead except that atrial capture

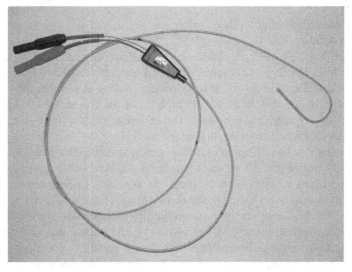

Figure 2.11 A standard "J-shaped" 5 French temporary atrial pacing wire.

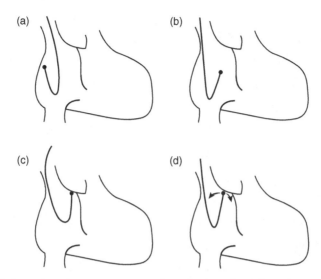

Figure 2.12 Insertion of a transvenous pacing wire into the right atrium. Panel (a) The pacing wire should be advanced into the right atrium as with a ventricular pacing wire. Panel (b) The tip of the wire should positioned anteriorly by applying torque and (c) the wire should be withdrawn until the tip is against the endocardium and slightly opened out. (d) Once in the correct position, the wire tip should rock from side to side with atrial contraction.

is confirmed by the presence of P waves following each pacing spike rather than QRS complexes. A dual chamber pacing box is required when atrial and ventricular leads are used (Figure 2.14). Pacing parameters for both leads can be set separately and different pacing modes can be programmed. In addition, the AV delay can be set manually, which can be useful to optimize cardiac output in patients with signs of heart failure.

Overdrive suppression of tachyarrhythmias using transvenous pacing wires

This technique requires routine pacing wire insertion as described above and a pacing box that can pace at high rates. Typically, such boxes have a switch or button (sometimes requiring a key to operate) that increases the pacing rate by a factor of three (Figure 2.15). This technique should only be used by experienced operators as pacing at high rates can lead to the development of AF or VF. The presence of a defibrillator next to the patient during the maneuver is mandatory. Typically, tachycardias arising from the atrium are terminated using atrial pacing in contrast to ventricular tachyarrhythmias, which are paced from the ventricle. However, there are important exceptions to this rule and specialist advice is essential before attempting this technique.

Pacing should be attempted at 10 bpm faster than the rate of the tachycardia and initially should be delivered in short bursts of up to eight beats.

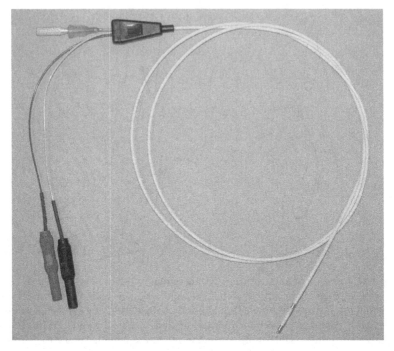

Figure 2.13 A standard 5 French "active-fixation" temporary pacing wire. The screw-in mechanism at the distal end (bottom, right) is controlled using the silver control (top left).

Failure to terminate tachycardia may occur because pacing has not captured the appropriate chamber (and therefore a higher voltage may be required) or the pacing rate is too slow, or a longer train of paced beats is required to achieve capture before stopping pacing. Thus, the voltage should be manipulated first before changing the pacing rate or duration. The pulse width (a feature that can be programmed on some pacing boxes) can also be increased to try to achieve capture. Manipulation of these settings will often lead to successful termination of the tachycardias described above and once termination is achieved, pacing at higher rates (e.g. 100 bpm) may prevent further episodes of tachycardia. If tachycardia continues to recur despite repeated successful overdrive pacing, further pharmacological therapy is probably indicated for which specialist advice should be sought.

External (transcutaneous) pacing
External pacing is available on most modern defibrillator units that are present in most A&E and Coronary Care Unit (CCU) departments for the emergency treatment of bradyarrhythmias, typically prior to transvenous pacing. An example of a defibrillator with external pacing facility is shown in Figure 2.16.

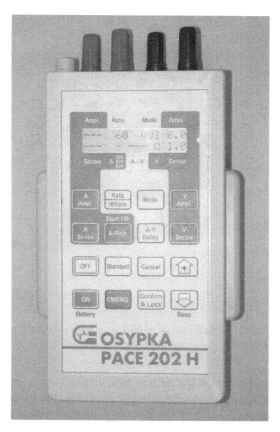

Figure 2.14 A standard dual chamber temporary pacing box. There are separate controls for atrial and ventricular pacing parameters as well as for pacing mode and AV delay.

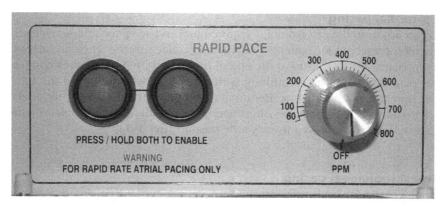

Figure 2.15 Controls for rapid overdrive pacing. On this model, the two red buttons on the left have to be pressed simultaneously to activate rapid pacing. The dial on the right is used to control the pacing rate.

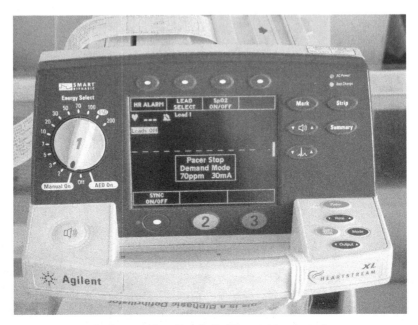

Figure 2.16 A standard external cardiac defibrillator with external, transcutaneous pacing facility. The buttons at the bottom right control pacing rate, mode, and output.

Adhesive pads are placed on the patient usually in an anteroposterior configuration and a current applied, which can be altered manually until ventricular capture occurs. This pacing technique is often uncomfortable for the patient, who may require sedation if pacing by this method is prolonged. It has been shown to be effective in 78–94% of patients for periods up to 14 hours.[27,28]

Epicardial pacing
Direct access to the epicardium is required for this pacing technique which is therefore reserved for patients undergoing cardiac surgery. They are placed prophylactically in theater at the end of the procedure. Fine wire electrodes are placed through the epicardium with connecting wires tunneled through the skin and to a pacing box. Because of their poor structural integrity, their pacing and sensing capabilities often deteriorates rapidly after initial placement and are typically removed using gentle traction after 3–5 days.

Transesophageal pacing
Both ventricular and atrial capture can be achieved using this technique although only the former is usually employed in the emergency setting. Some studies have shown this pacing route to be better tolerated than transcutaneous pacing.[29]

Table 2.2 Complications of temporary transvenous cardiac pacing

Acute complications

Complications arising from venous access
  1 Pneumothorax
  2 Hemothorax
  3 Inadvertent arterial puncture

Complications arising from initial placement of pacing lead
  1 Temporary or sustained episodes of ventricular ectopy
  2 Cardiac perforation and tamponade
  3 Diaphragmatic pacing

Complications arising following placement of pacing lead
  1 Sudden failure to capture
    (a) Oversensing
    (b) Movement of the lead
    (c) Dislodged connections

Subacute complications
  1 Infection

Complications of temporary pacing

Acute and subacute complications arising from transvenous cardiac pacing are shown in Table 2.2. Venous access can be complicated by hemorrhage, pneumothorax or hemothorax, or inadvertent arterial puncture. Selecting the jugular route may minimize this risk.

Placement of the pacing wire can lead to temporary or sustained episodes of ventricular ectopy, which has been dealt with above. Once capture has been achieved, patients may rapidly become pacing dependent (i.e. abrupt cessation of pacing will lead to asystole) and if repositioning is required in this setting, pacing should be weaned off gradually by reducing the rate slowly until an underlying rhythm is identified.

As mentioned above, cardiac perforation can occur especially with the lead at the extreme RVA and can lead to cardiac tamponade. Prior to this, a rise in pacing threshold or the presence of pericardial chest pain, dyspnea, or a pericardial rub should alert the clinician to the possibility of perforation and echocardiography should be performed urgently. If present, withdrawal of the lead back to the endocardium usually corrects the problem although this can occasionally precipitate tamponade.

Failure to achieve a pacing threshold <1 V is common in patients with extensive inferior infarction, cardiomyopathies, or those on Class I antiarrhythmic drugs, and higher thresholds can be accepted. In addition, the pacing threshold typically doubles within 24 h of lead placement due the development of local edema. Daily testing of each wire to determine the capture threshold is therefore mandatory. However, a rising threshold or intermittent loss of capture should lead to consideration of lead repositioning.

Sudden failure to capture should alert the clinician to the possibility of over-sensing and the sensitivity should be reduced or fixed-rate pacing (VOO mode) employed to diagnose the problem. In addition, all connections should be checked thoroughly and the batteries in the pacing box replaced if necessary. If capture is still not achieved, the voltage should be increased prior to urgent repositioning of the wire.

Diaphragmatic pacing is usually only seen with high voltages (or may be seen with perforation) and the voltage should be reduced if capture can still be obtained or if not, the wire repositioned.

Longer-term complications include infection, and the sheath site should be examined daily for signs of inflammation or pus. When present, replace-ment of the wire is almost always required (through a different access point) and this may delay progression to permanent pacing, if indicated. There-fore, temporary pacing wires should be removed as rapidly as possible and a permanent system implanted, if indicated. If this is not possible, temporary wires should be changed electively after 7 days by a new puncture and wire to limit the risk of local and systemic infection. Prophylactic antibiotics are not routinely employed unless obtaining vascular access has been unusually difficult.

Thrombus can form on the wire and lead to thromboembolic complications, especially using the femoral route. For this reason in some centers, patients are routinely heparinized (unless contraindications exist), especially if using the femoral route in an emergency.

Conclusion

Temporary cardiac pacing is now a standard treatment for patients with symp-tomatic bradycardia, heart block, and several types of tachyarrhythmia. It has become an integral part of acute cardiac care, often acting as a bridging ther-apy prior to permanent pacing. Physicians and cardiac-care personnel should be familiar with its indications and implantation techniques, and should be aware of potential hazards and problems that may be encountered in the after care of patients undergoing temporary pacing.

References

1 Zoll PM. Resuscitation of the heart in ventricular standstill by external electric stimulation. *N Engl J Med* 1952; 247: 768–71.
2 Furman S, Robinson G. The use of an intracardiac pacemaker in the correction of total heart block. *Surg Forum* 1958; 9: 245–8.
3 Furman S, Robinson G. Stimulation of the ventricular endocardial surface in control of complete heart block. *Ann Surg* 1959; 150: 841–5.

4 Waldo AL, MacLean WA, Karp RB *et al.* Continuous rapid atrial pacing to control recurrent or sustained supraventricular tachycardias following open heart surgery. *Circulation* 1976; 54: 245–50.

5 Cooper TB, MacLean WA, Waldo AL. Overdrive pacing for supraventricular tachycardia: a review of theoretical implications and therapeutic techniques. *Pacing Clin Electrophysiol* 1978; 1: 196–221.

6 Calvo RA, Saksena S, Pantopoulos D. Sequential transvenous pacing and shock therapy for termination of sustained ventricular tachycardia. *Am Heart J* 1988; 115: 569–75.

7 Estes NA, III, Deering TF, Manolis AS *et al.* External cardiac programmed stimulation for noninvasive termination of sustained supraventricular and ventricular tachycardia. *Am J Cardiol* 1989; 63: 177–83.

8 Volkmann H, Dannberg G, Heinke M *et al.* Termination of tachycardias by transesophageal electrical pacing. *Pacing Clin Electrophysiol* 1992; 15: 1962–6.

9 Ryan TJ, Antman EM, Brooks NH *et al.* 1999 update: ACC/AHA Guidelines for the Management of Patients With Acute Myocardial Infarction: Executive Summary and Recommendations: a report of the American College of Cardiology/American Heart Association Task Force on Practice Guidelines (Committee on Management of Acute Myocardial Infarction). *Circulation* 1999; 100: 1016–30.

10 Aplin M, Engstrom T, Vejlstrup NG *et al.* Prognostic importance of complete atrioventricular block complicating acute myocardial infarction. *Am J Cardiol* 2003; 92: 853–6.

11 Sanchez-Quintana D, Ho SY, Cabrera JA *et al.* Topographic anatomy of the inferior pyramidal space: relevance to radiofrequency catheter ablation. *J Cardiovasc Electrophysiol* 2001; 12: 210–17.

12 Barold SS, Hayes DL. Second-degree atrioventricular block: a reappraisal. *Mayo Clin Proc* 2001; 76: 44–57.

13 Ferez S, Guizar S, Cardenas M. The Wenckebach phenomenon in patients with acute myocardial infarction. *Arch Inst Cardiol Mex* 1988; 58: 209–214.

14 Lamas GA. Physiological consequences of normal atrioventricular conduction: applicability to modern cardiac pacing. *J Card Surg* 1989; 4: 89–98.

15 Samet P, Castillo C, Bernstein WH. Hemodynamic consequences of atrial and ventricular pacing in subjects with normal hearts. *Am J Cardiol* 1966; 18: 522–5.

16 Rahimtoola SH, Ehsani A, Sinno MZ *et al.* Left atrial transport function in myocardial infarction. Importance of its booster pump function. *Am J Med* 1975; 59: 686–94.

17 Boucher CA, Pohost GM, Okada RD *et al.* Effect of ventricular pacing on left ventricular function assessed by radionuclide angiography. *Am Heart J* 1983; 106: 1105–11.

18 Murphy P, Morton P, Murtagh JG *et al.* Hemodynamic effects of different temporary pacing modes for the management of bradycardias complicating acute myocardial infarction. *Pacing Clin Electrophysiol* 1992; 15: 391–6.

19 Connolly SJ, Kerr CR, Gent M *et al.* Effects of physiologic pacing versus ventricular pacing on the risk of stroke and death due to cardiovascular causes. Canadian Trial of Physiologic Pacing Investigators. *N Engl J Med* 2000; 342: 1385–91.

20 Lamas GA, Lee KL, Sweeney MO *et al.* Ventricular pacing or dual-chamber pacing for sinus-node dysfunction. *N Engl J Med* 2002; 346: 1854–62.

21 Mamiya K, Aono J, Manabe M. Complete atrioventricular block during anesthesia. *Can J Anaesth* 1999; 46: 265–7.

22 Gauss A, Hubner C, Meierhenrich R *et al.* Perioperative transcutaneous pacemaker in patients with chronic bifascicular block or left bundle branch block and additional first-degree atrioventricular block. *Acta Anaesthesiol Scand* 1999; 43: 731–6.

23 Gauss A, Hubner C, Radermacher P *et al.* Perioperative risk of bradyarrhythmias in patients with asymptomatic chronic bifascicular block or left bundle branch block: does an additional first-degree atrioventricular block make any difference? *Anesthesiology* 1998; 88: 679–87.

24 Mikell FL, Weir EK, Chesler E. Perioperative risk of complete heart block in patients with bifascicular block and prolonged PR interval. *Thorax* 1981; 36: 14–17.

25 Pastore JO, Yurchak PM, Janis KM *et al.* The risk of advanced heart block in surgical patients with right bundle branch block and left axis deviation. *Circulation* 1978; 57: 677–80.

26 Venkataraman K, Madias JE, Hood WB, Jr. Indications for prophylactic preoperative insertion of pacemakers in patients with right bundle branch block and left anterior hemiblock. *Chest* 1975; 68: 501–6.

27 Madsen JK, Meibom J, Videbak R *et al.* Transcutaneous pacing: experience with the Zoll noninvasive temporary pacemaker. *Am Heart J* 1988; 116: 7–10.

28 Zoll PM, Zoll RH, Falk RH *et al.* External noninvasive temporary cardiac pacing: clinical trials. *Circulation* 1985; 71: 937–44.

29 McEneaney DJ, Cochrane DJ, Anderson JA *et al.* Ventricular pacing with a novel gastroesophageal electrode: a comparison with external pacing. *Am Heart J* 1997; 133: 674–80.

CHAPTER 3

Pacemaker implantation and indications

Aneesh V. Tolat and Peter J. Zimetbaum

Indications

Pacemakers are implanted to alleviate symptoms and/or prevent subsequent morbidity or mortality that may result from bradycardia. Bradycardia can result from a variety of disorders of the sinus node, the atrioventricular (AV) node, the His-Purkinje system, or of a combination of these. Sinus node or AV nodal disease is often not life threatening, but may cause significant symptoms. On the other hand, disease of the His-Purkinje system may be asymptomatic until the development of serious adverse events.

Symptoms from bradycardia generally result from diminished cardiac output. Such symptoms may be vague and include fatigue, decreased exercise tolerance, dyspnea on exertion, light-headedness, dizziness, congestive heart failure, presyncope, or syncope. Other symptoms, such as neck pulsation, may be related to AV dyssynchrony, resulting in intermittent forceful atrial contraction against a closed tricuspid valve (this physical sign is known as "cannon A waves"). Patient-triggered ambulatory cardiac monitoring is often helpful in establishing that symptoms, which may be nonspecific, are in fact the result of symptomatic bradycardia. Tables 3.1–3.5 summarize some of the more common indications for permanent cardiac pacing published by the American College of Cardiology/American Heart Association Task Force on Practice Guidelines in 2002.[1–3] Terminology used in the guidelines and by some cardiologists and electrophysiologists is discussed below.

New Class I indications for permanent pacing in the 2002 guidelines include: advanced second-degree AV block, heart failure as a major symptom from AV block induced bradycardia, patients with neuromuscular disease with third-degree AV block (regardless of the presence of symptoms), alternating bundle branch block (BBB), and congenital third-degree AV block with complex ventricular ectopy. Some electrocardiogram (ECG) examples of AV block and sinus node dysfunction requiring permanent pacemaker implantation are shown in Figures 3.1–3.3. In addition, an example of pacemaker inhibition is shown in Figure 3.4 (see figure and text on VVI pacing mode for more details).

Table 3.1 The 2002 recommendations for permanent pacing in acquired AV block in adults

---

Class I

1. Third-degree and advanced second-degree AV block at any anatomic level, associated with any one of the following conditions:
   (a) Bradycardia with symptoms (including heart failure) presumed to be due to AV block.
   (b) Arrhythmias and other medical conditions that require drugs that result in symptomatic bradycardia.
   (c) Documented periods of asystole ≥3.0 s or any escape rate less than 40 beats per minute (bpm) in awake, symptom-free patients.
   (d) After catheter ablation of the AV junction. There are no trials to assess outcomes without pacing, and pacing is virtually always planned in this situation unless the operative procedure is AV junction modification.
   (e) Postoperative AV block that is not expected to resolve after cardiac surgery.
   (f) Neuromuscular diseases with AV block, such as myotonic muscular dystrophy, Kearns–Sayre syndrome, Erb's dystrophy (limb-girdle), and peroneal muscular atrophy, with or without symptoms, because there may be unpredictable progression of AV conduction disease.

Class IIa

1. Asymptomatic third-degree AV block at any anatomic site with average awake ventricular rates of 40 bpm or faster especially if cardiomegaly or left ventricular (LV) dysfunction is present.
2. Asymptomatic Type II second-degree AV block with a narrow QRS. When Type II second-degree AV block occurs with a wide QRS, pacing becomes a Class I recommendation (see the section regarding Pacing for chronic bifascicular and trifascicular block).
3. Asymptomatic Type I second-degree AV block at intra- or infra-His levels found at electrophysiological study performed for other indications.
4. First- or second-degree AV block with symptoms similar to those of pacemaker syndrome.

Class IIb

1. Marked first-degree AV block (more than 0.30 s) in patients with LV dysfunction and symptoms of congestive heart failure in whom a shorter AV interval results in hemodynamic improvement, presumably by decreasing left atrial filling pressure.
2. Neuromuscular diseases such as myotonic muscular dystrophy, Kearns-Sayre syndrome, Erb's dystrophy (limb-girdle), and peroneal muscular atrophy with any degree of AV block (including first-degree AV block) with or without symptoms, because there may be unpredictable progression of AV conduction disease.

Class III

1. Asymptomatic first-degree AV block. (See also "Pacing for chronic bifascicular and trifascicular block")
2. Asymptomatic Type I second-degree AV block at the supra-His (AV node) level or not known to be intra- or infra-Hisian.
3. AV block expected to resolve and/or unlikely to recur (e.g. drug toxicity, Lyme disease, or during hypoxia in sleep apnea syndrome in absence of symptoms).

Note: Class I – there is evidence and/or general agreement that a pacemaker is beneficial/useful/effective. Class II – conflicting evidence and/or opinion. Class IIa – weight of evidence/opinion is in favor of usefulness/efficacy. Class IIb – efficacy of pacemaker is less well established. Class III – evidence and/or general agreement that pacemaker is not useful and may be harmful.

Advanced second-degree AV block refers to AV block that is more than AV Wenckebach, and usually implies intermittent AV conduction that may not fall into the category of second-degree Type II AV block.

Source: Adapted from the ACC/AHA/NASPE 2002 guideline update.[1–3]

Table 3.2 The 2002 recommendations for permanent pacing in chronic bifascicular and trifascicular block

---

Class I

1. Intermittent third-degree AV block.
2. Type II second-degree AV block.
3. Alternating bundle branch block.

Class IIa

1. Syncope not demonstrated to be due to AV block when other likely causes have been excluded, specifically ventricular tachycardia (VT).
2. Incidental finding at electrophysiological study or markedly prolonged HV interval (≥100 ms) in asymptomatic patients.
3. Incidental finding at electrophysiological study of pacing-induced infra-His block that is not physiological.

Class IIb

1. Neuromuscular diseases such as myotonic muscular dystrophy, Kearns–Sayre syndrome, Erb's dystrophy (limb-girdle), and peroneal muscular atrophy with any degree of fascicular block with or without symptoms, because there may be unpredictable progression of AV conduction disease.

Class III

1. Fascicular block without AV block or symptoms.
2. Fascicular block with first-degree AV block without symptoms.

Note: Class I – there is evidence and/or general agreement that a pacemaker is beneficial/useful/effective. Class II – conflicting evidence and/or opinion. Class IIa – weight of evidence/opinion is in favor of usefulness/efficacy. Class IIb – efficacy of pacemaker is less well established. Class III – evidence and/or general agreement that pacemaker is not useful and may be harmful.

Source: Adapted from the ACC/AHA/NASPE 2002 guideline update.[1–3]

Growth in pacemaker use

With an aging worldwide population, the number of patients requiring implantation of pacemakers for sinus node dysfunction and AV block is expected to continue increasing. Figure 3.6 shows the yearly growth in the number of pacemakers for the United States over the past 40 years. Since 2002, analysts estimate that over 250 000 pacemakers have been implanted per year in the United States, with a similar number of pacemakers implanted in Europe.[4] Based on data from previous years, about 50% or more of pacemakers are implanted for sinus node dysfunction.[5,6] The number of pacemakers implanted in the future may be offset by implantable cardioverter-defibrillators that are increasingly being used for primary prevention of sudden cardiac death.

Pacemaker nomenclature

The nomenclature for describing pacemaker function has evolved significantly since their creation and reflects the increasing functions that they are

Table 3.3 The 2002 recommendations for permanent pacing in sinus node dysfunction

---

Class I

1. Sinus node dysfunction with documented symptomatic bradycardia, including frequent sinus pauses that produce symptoms. In some patients, bradycardia is iatrogenic and will occur as a consequence of essential long-term drug therapy of a type and dose for which there are no acceptable alternatives.
2. Symptomatic chronotropic incompetence.

Class IIa

1. Sinus node dysfunction occurring spontaneously or as a result of necessary drug therapy, with heart rate less than 40 bpm when a clear association between significant symptoms consistent with bradycardia and the actual presence of bradycardia has not been documented.
2. Syncope of unexplained origin when major abnormalities of sinus node function are discovered or provoked in electrophysiological studies.

Class IIb

1. In minimally symptomatic patients, chronic heart rate less than 40 bpm while awake.

Class III

1. Sinus node dysfunction in asymptomatic patients, including those in whom substantial sinus bradycardia (heart rate less than 40 bpm) is a consequence of long-term drug treatment.
2. Sinus node dysfunction in patients with symptoms suggestive of bradycardia that are clearly documented as not associated with a slow heart rate.
3. Sinus node dysfunction with symptomatic bradycardia due to nonessential drug therapy.

Note: Class I – there is evidence and/or general agreement that a pacemaker is beneficial/useful/effective. Class II – conflicting evidence and/or opinion. Class IIa – weight of evidence/opinion is in favor of usefulness/efficacy. Class IIb – efficacy of pacemaker is less well established. Class III – evidence and/or general agreement that pacemaker is not useful and may be harmful.
Source: Adapted from the ACC/AHA/NASPE 2002 guideline update.[1–3]

capable of providing. The current nomenclature was established by the North American Society of Pacing and Electrophysiology (NASPE/Heart Rhythm Society) and the British Pacing and Electrophysiology Group (BPEG) and is referred to as the NBG code[7] (Table 3.6). The code allows for five letters, though 3–4 letters are used most commonly.

The first letter designates the chamber or chambers paced: A = atrium; V = ventricle; and D = dual chamber (both atrium and ventricle). The second letter indicates the chamber or chambers in which sensing occurs. The letters used (A, V, D) are the same as above. The third letter indicates the response to a sensed event. In this position the letters used are: I = inhibit; T = triggered; and D = dual *response* (both inhibited and triggered), which is only possible for dual chamber pacemakers. For example, in a single chamber pacemaker with an "I" in the third position, a sensed event by a ventricular lead would

Table 3.4 The 2002 recommendations for permanent pacing after the acute phase of myocardial infarction

---

Class I

1. Persistent second-degree AV block in the His-Purkinje system with bilateral bundle branch block or third-degree AV block within or below the His-Purkinje system after acute myocardial infarction (AMI).
2. Transient advanced (second- or third-degree) infranodal AV block and associated bundle branch block. If the site of block is uncertain, an electrophysiological study may be necessary.
3. Persistent and symptomatic second- or third-degree AV block.

Class IIb

1. Persistent second- or third-degree AV block at the AV node level.

Class III

1. Transient AV block in the absence of intraventricular conduction defects.
2. Transient AV block in the presence of isolated left anterior fascicular block.
3. Acquired left anterior fascicular block in the absence of AV block.
4. Persistent first-degree AV block in the presence of bundle branch block that is old or age indeterminate.

Note: Class I – there is evidence and/or general agreement that a pacemaker is beneficial/useful/effective. Class II – conflicting evidence and/or opinion. Class IIa – weight of evidence/opinion is in favor of usefulness/efficacy. Class IIb – efficacy of pacemaker is less well established. Class III – evidence and/or general agreement that pacemaker is not useful and may be harmful.
Source: Adapted from the ACC/AHA/NASPE 2002 guideline update.[1–3]

prevent the pacemaker from delivering a stimulus in the ventricle following the sensed event for a prespecified period of time. However, with a "T" in the third position, a sensed event in the ventricle would *trigger* a paced beat in the ventricle. In patients with dual chamber pacemakers, a "D" is also possible. In this case, a sensed event in the atrium could inhibit atrial stimulation and also trigger delivery of a paced beat in the ventricle.

The fourth position in the code is used to specify whether the pacemaker has additional programmability such as rate modulation. Rate modulation implies that the pacemaker has a sensor that can increase the paced rate based on the sensor's ability to recognize an increase in motion or respiration. The letter "R" in the fourth position denotes the capability of the pacemaker to provide this function. The other programming functions and letters for this position are shown in the accompanying table but are not commonly used.

Finally, the fifth position was created to describe location or absence of multisite pacing. In this case, "A" would indicate multisite pacing in the atrium, a "V" would indicate multisite pacing in the ventricle, and "D" would indicate multisite pacing in the atrium and ventricle. For practical purposes, the fifth letter is rarely used, though with the advent of biventricular pacing (BVP) this may change.

Table 3.5 The 2002 recommendations for permanent pacing in hypersensitive carotid sinus syndrome and neurocardiogenic syncope

---

Class I

1. Recurrent syncope caused by carotid sinus stimulation; minimal carotid sinus pressure induces ventricular asystole of more than 3-s duration in the absence of any medication that depresses the sinus node or AV conduction.

Class IIa

1. Recurrent syncope without clear, provocative events and with a hypersensitive cardioinhibitory response.
2. Syncope of unexplained origin when major abnormalities of sinus node function or AV conduction are discovered or provoked in electrophysiological studies.
3. Significantly symptomatic and recurrent neurocardiogenic syncope associated with bradycardia documented spontaneously or at the time of tilt-table testing.

Class IIb

1. Neurally mediated syncope with significant bradycardia reproduced by a head-up tilt with or without isoproterenol or other provocative maneuvers.

Class III

1. A hyperactive cardioinhibitory response to carotid sinus stimulation in the absence of symptoms or in the presence of vague symptoms such as dizziness, lightheadedness, or both.
2. A hyperactive cardioinhibitory response to carotid sinus stimulation in the presence of vague symptoms such as dizziness, lightheadedness, or both.
3. Recurrent syncope, lightheadedness, or dizziness in the absence of a hyperactive cardioinihibitory response.
4. Situational vasovagal syncope in which avoidance behavior is effective.

Note: Class I – there is evidence and/or general agreement that a pacemaker is beneficial/useful/effective. Class II – conflicting evidence and/or opinion. Class IIa – weight of evidence/opinion is in favor of usefulness/efficacy. Class IIb – efficacy of pacemaker is less well established. Class III – evidence and/or general agreement that pacemaker is not useful and may be harmful.
Source: Adapted from the ACC/AHA/NASPE 2002 guideline update.[1–3]

Modes

Choosing a particular pacing mode for the individual patient can sometimes be confusing for the less experienced. In general, the patient's cardiac and related medical conditions determine what mode might be best for a particular patient. For example, does the patient have a normal or reduced ejection fraction (EF)? Does the patient have normal or abnormal conduction? The number of leads connected to the pulse generator also determines how many pacing mode options will be available.

Single chamber pacing

Single chamber pacing (AAI and VVI) is usually reserved for patients with only one lead either in the atrium or ventricle. In these modes, only atrial or

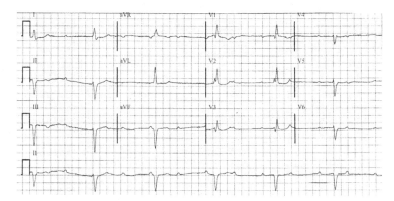

Figure 3.1 ECG of an 88-year-old man with a 1 week history of fatigue and dyspnea. The escape rhythm at 35 bpm, shows a QRS with right BBB, left anterior fascicular block morphology. In this case the bifascicular block was known previously implying that the escape rhythm originates above the site of bifascicular block. The patient received a dual chamber pacemaker with improvement in symptoms. Bifascicular block implies block in two of three of the fascicles/ bundle (right bundle, left anterior fascicle, and left posterior fascicle) that carry electrical impulses from the His bundle to the ventricles. The left bundle branch is made up of the left anterior fascicle and the left posterior fascicle. Trifascicular block implies block in both the left anterior and left posterior fascicles that make up the left bundle as well as the right bundle.

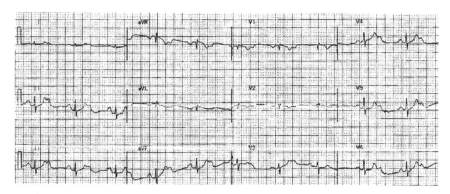

Figure 3.2 Stress test ECG obtained during stress testing in a 65-year-old physician with complaints of dyspnea during exercise. His resting ECG showed normal 1 : 1 AV conduction. However, during exertion he was noted to have 2 : 1 AV block that was responsible for a decreased cardiac output and his symptoms. He underwent dual chamber pacemaker implantation with dramatic improvement in his symptoms during exercise.

ventricular pacing and sensing in the respective chamber are possible. While the pacemaker can still be programmed to have rate-responsive modulation by a sensor (which can detect when a patient may be exercising and require an increase in the heart rate), it will be independent of the other chamber. The

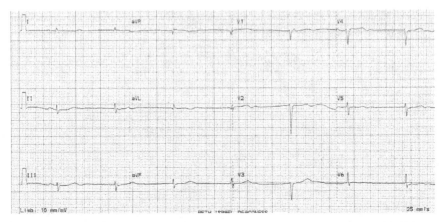

Figure 3.3 ECG of a 72-year-old man with recent conversion from AF on dofetilide. The figure shows one sinus beat (far left) followed by a junctional escape rhythm with sinus arrest. Note the long QT interval associated with bradycardia. The patient continued to have sinus arrest and subsequently underwent pacemaker implantation.

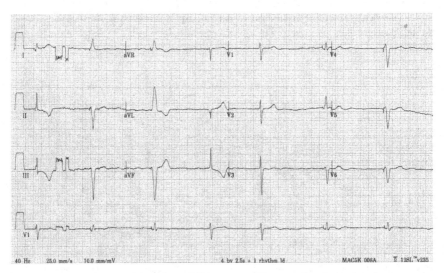

Figure 3.4 Example of pacemaker inhibition. In this example, the patient's pacemaker is set to a backup pacing rate of 45 bpm. Looking at the rhythm strip in V1, beats #2 and #3 are paced beats because the patients intrinsic ventricular rhythm was slower than 45 bpm. However, when the intrinsic ventricular rhythm accelerates to >45 bpm, as in beats #4 and #5, the pacemaker is inhibited.

response to a sensed event in the chamber with the lead is inhibition of the pacemaker. As a result of the inhibition function, a lower rate limit needs to be specified so that the pacemaker knows how long to wait prior to delivering a pacing stimulus. For VVI pacemakers, if in that period of time a sensed

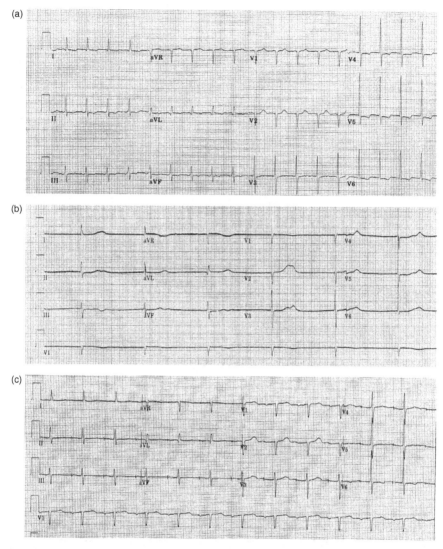

Figure 3.5 Three panels of ECGs are shown of a patient who presented with palpitations and was found to have an atrial tachycardia (a). She was started on a β blocker and then developed symptoms of light-headedness and dizziness and was found to have sinus arrest with a junctional escape rhythm (b). Her β blocker was held, and she underwent implantation of a dual chamber pacemaker (c) followed by resumption of her β blocker.

event occurs in the ventricle, then the pacemaker is inhibited (see Figure 3.4). However, if no sensed event occurs in that time period, then the pacemaker delivers a pacing stimulus in the ventricle. The primary disadvantage of this mode is a lack of AV synchrony during ventricular pacing.

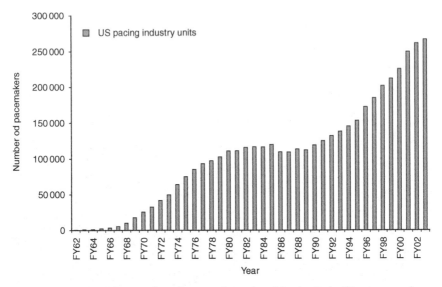

Figure 3.6 Graph of the number of pacemakers placed in the United States over the past 40 years.[4] (Courtesy of Medtronic.)

Table 3.6 Revised NBG code for pacing nomenclature

Position	I	II	III	IV	V
Category	Chamber(s) paced	Chamber(s) sensed	Response to sensing	Rate modulation	Multisite pacing
	0=none	0=none	0=none	0=none	0=none
	A=atrium	A=atrium	T=triggered	R=rate modulation	A=atrium
	V=ventricle	V=ventricle	I=inhibited		V=ventricle
	D=dual	D=dual	D=dual		D=dual
	(A+V)	(A+V)	(T+I)		(A+V)

Source: Adapted from Bernstein AD, Daubert JC, Fletcher RD *et al*. The revised NASPE/BPEG generic code for antibradycardia, adaptive-rate, and multisite pacing. North American Society of Pacing and Electrophysiology/British Pacing and Electrophysiology Group. *Pacing Clin Electrophysiol* 2002; 25: 260–4.

The AAI mode is similar to the VVI mode except that the chamber in which the lead paces and senses is the atrium. This mode is not generally seen in the United States because most pacemaker implants that incorporate a lead in the atrium also include a lead in the ventricle. In the majority of cases this is done so that future AV conduction disturbances do not require the patient to undergo a second procedure in order to place a second lead. The AAI mode, like the VVI mode, allows for atrial pacing and sensing. A sensed atrial event within a specified time period leads to inhibition of the pacemaker. The AAI mode, though uncommon, is used primarily for patients with sinus node dysfunction. The primary disadvantage in this mode would be the inability to pace the ventricle and maintain hemodynamic stability should heart block occur without a stable escape rhythm. The frequency with which this occurs is thought to be in the order of <1% per year.[8]

Dual chamber pacing

Dual chamber AV pacing is possible when one lead is present in the atrium and one lead is present in the ventricle. The two most commonly used pacing modes are DDD and DDI. These modes allow for pacing and sensing in both the atrium and the ventricle. The key difference comes from the response that each mode has to a sensed event. The DDD mode allows for *dual* or triggered and inhibited responses to a sensed event. Hence atrial or ventricular pacing in DDD mode can be inhibited by a sensed event in either chamber. In addition, the ventricular pacing lead can be used to deliver a pacing stimulus (trigger) in the ventricle after a sensed event in the atrium, after a specified period of time. The advantage of this mode is that AV synchrony can be maintained. However, during atrial tachyarrhythmias, the ventricle will be stimulated to pace and maintain AV synchrony at a rate up to or equal to the programmed upper rate limit of the pacemaker. Though this may be a significant problem, newer pacemakers have the additional ability to change modes during an atrial tachyarrhythmia (DDD to VVI) known as "mode switching" or "atrial tachycardia response." The programmed DDD pacemaker has the ability to recognize atrial arrhythmias and change modes so that the ventricle is not forced to rapid atrial rates inappropriately. This is particularly useful in patients with a history of atrial tachycardia, atrial flutter, or fibrillation. If this is not available, then the patient's pacemaker should be programmed to DDI mode. These changes in mode have been used as a surrogate marker of atrial tachyarrhythmias and more specifically atrial fibrillation (AF). One additional small disadvantage of the DDD mode involves the possibility that pacemaker-mediated tachycardia (PMT) can occur. PMT occurs when a ventricular ectopic beat leads to atrial depolarization via retrograde (ventriculoatrial) conduction. If this atrial depolarization occurs outside the PVARP (post ventriculo atrial refractory period), the pacemaker recognizes (senses) it and allows the ventricle to track the atrial depolarization, thus setting up an endless loop, or PMT.

In DDI mode, the pacemaker can only be *inhibited* from delivering a pacing stimulus in either chamber. Unlike DDD, this mode does not allow the pacemaker to pace the ventricle after a sensed event in the atrium and "track" the atrial rate. During only ventricular pacing, AV dyssynchrony can occur leading to "pacemaker syndrome" in which the atrium contracts against a closed tricuspid valve leading to "cannon A waves" and regurgitant blood flow into the jugular veins. In this mode, AV synchrony will only be maintained when there is native AV conduction or pacing in both the atrium and ventricle.

Unlike DDD, in the DDI mode atrial tachyarrhythmias will not lead to inappropriately high paced ventricular rates. The advantage of DDI mode is that in patients who need almost no ventricular pacing, native AV conduction is allowed to occur with sparing of battery life.

Other modes that have been used in the past include VDD and DVI. The DVI mode was used largely because of the limitation of available technology. By definition, in the DVI mode, pacemakers can pace both the atrium and ventricle, and sense only in the ventricle. As a result, the ventricle can be paced when no activity is present for a prespecified time period. The pacemaker is however limited to pacing the ventricle without AV synchrony. In addition, since pacing but not sensing can occur in the atrium, pacing in the atrium may occur in addition to native atrial activity, which may lead to atrial tachyarrhythmias.

The VDD mode has been used in single lead systems that have a proximal sensor to identify atrial activity and a distal electrode for both sensing and pacing in the ventricle. The advantage of this mode is that it allows for a single lead pacemaker to pace the ventricle and yet maintain AV synchrony by tracking the atrium. Unfortunately, the disadvantage of this mode involves potential problems with positioning of the atrial chamber electrode. If the electrode is not in a stable location, then there can be a failure to sense atrial activity.

Mode and device selection

Choosing a particular pacemaker and particular mode depends on the patient's underlying medical condition, health of the sinus node and native AV conduction, as well as EF. Most patients can be divided into those with sinus node dysfunction and those with AV conduction disturbances.

Sinus node dysfunction

For those patients with only sinus node dysfunction and intact AV conduction, a single lead placed in the atrium with the pacemaker programmed AAI would ordinarily suffice for treating the patient's bradycardia. However, as noted earlier, at least in the United States, while theoretically pacing only the atrium makes sense, standard practice has been to implant pacemakers with one lead in the atrium and one lead in the ventricle. In these patients, with a dual chamber pacemaker and only sinus node dysfunction, either DDIR or DDDR pacing modes would be appropriate. Rate modulation (the fourth letter "R") would be useful to add to either the DDI or DDD pacing modes, since these patients by definition have abnormal sinus node function. The DDIR mode is preferred if there is no need for ventricular pacing because it will conserve battery life. Recent data from the Dual Chamber and VVI Implantable Defibrillator Trial (DAVID) demonstrated an increase in the incidence of congestive heart failure associated with right ventricular (RV) pacing.[9] This potential complication of obligatory RV pacing represents another compelling indication for DDIR pacing. While patients in this trial also had left ventricular systolic dysfunction, the concept of avoiding RV pacing can be generalized to patients with normal EFs.

The VVI mode appears to have a lesser role in patients with sinus node dysfunction. In the Mode Selection Trial (MOST), a comparison of dual chamber versus single chamber VVI pacing in patients with sinus node dysfunction, VVI pacing was associated with a higher risk for AF, signs and symptoms of congestive heart failure, and poorer quality of life scores.[10] It should be noted that in MOST, patients with dual chamber pacing and a narrow normal QRS without pacing were more likely to be at risk for heart failure hospitalizations as well as the recurrence of AF, implying that pacing can be detrimental in patients with a narrow QRS.[11] Another study also evaluated the role of pacemaker mode in patients with sinus node dysfunction and AV block. The Pacemaker Selection in the Elderly Investigators showed that there was a slight beneficial effect in clinical symptoms when using a dual chamber pacemaker for sinus node dysfunction whereas there was no meaningful difference in symptoms between single and dual chamber pacing in patients with AV block.[12] In addition, 26% of patients (patients with either sinus node dysfunction or AV block) assigned to ventricular pacing developed pacemaker syndrome and were reprogrammed to dual chamber pacing. Thus, in patients with sinus node dysfunction who have undergone pacemaker implantation, the use of dual chamber pacing appears to be the best approach as supported by the data above.

AV block

Patients with AV block can have either a single or dual chamber pacemaker implanted unless they have a history of chronic AF, which makes the presence of an atrial lead unnecessary. In patients with an intact sinus node and largely intact AV conduction and rare intermittent AV block, the VVI, DDI, DDD, and VDD pacing modes could be considered potential modes for pacing. The advantage of the dual chamber pacing mode is that it would potentially allow for more AV synchronous pacing. However, this may not be as important in the older patient in whom a single chamber pacemaker may suffice.[12,13] Data from the UKPACE (United Kingdom Pacing and Cardiovascular Events) trial as well as as from the Pacemaker Selection in the Elderly Investigators showed that in elderly patients (>65 years of age), single chamber pacing for patients with AV block was not associated with any adverse outcomes or symptoms. Given the technical ease of implantation of a single chamber pacemaker and the associated cost savings, one can promote the case for the use of single chamber pacing in the older patient. This form of pacing has not been evaluated in patients <65 years of age who are likely to be more sensitive to the loss of AV synchrony. In these patients with rare intermittent AV block, the DDI/R or DDD/R modes would be the best choice as discussed previously (see discussion in sinus node section).

In patients of <65 years of age who have less intact AV conduction and a normal sinus node, DDI/R pacing would be less worthwhile since the patient will be more likely to require pacing of the ventricle without the maintenance of AV synchrony. This can lead to cannon A waves, patient symptoms, and less efficient filling of the ventricle. In this situation, DDD/R pacing affords the best pacing option for the patient to allow AV synchrony. VDD pacing with a single lead is also feasible but requires the use of a special lead with an atrial electrode that is positioned in the atrium while placing the lead tip in the right ventricle. This would provide a result similar to DDD pacing but with the convenience of placing only a single lead. This, however, should only be considered in patients with normal sinus node function and should be weighed against the possibility of an unstable atrial electrode position (as mentioned earlier in the chapter).

As in patients with sinus node dysfunction, synchronizing the atrium and ventricle in patients with AV block is preferred over activating the atrium and ventricle dyssynchronously. However, the maintenance of AV synchrony comes at the cost of potentially creating intra- and interventricular dyssynchrony (see above). With the advent of BVP, this has become an area of intense interest and research. In patients with ventricular dyssynchrony, BVP may offer some benefit and should also be considered. However, some patients with prolonged AV conduction but not block may also in the future benefit from "physiologic pacing." Nonpacing modes are in development and have showed that by allowing for dynamic prolongation of the AV interval at faster atrial rates (minimal V pacing or "MVP"), AV synchrony can be maintained in DDD mode with a reduction in ventricular pacing.[14,15]

Special situations

Two special situations that have been used to justify pacemaker implantation deserve special mention. Vasovagal, or neurocardiogenic, syncope is caused by activation of a complex vagal reflex leading to a drop in blood pressure sometimes associated with significant bradycardia. Investigators have postulated that patients with significant bradycardia during their vagal syncope might benefit from the implantation of a pacemaker. Small unblinded trials showed potential benefit of pacemaker implantation in patients with vasovagal syncope.[16–18] Recently, the Second Vasovagal Pacemaker Study (VPS II), a blinded larger trial of pacemaker implantation for vasovagal syncope showed no significant benefit was derived from the implantation of a pacemaker.[19] Unfortunately, not enough patients with significant bradycardia (heart rate <40 bpm) or asystole were included in the trial to make a conclusion about the lack of effect of a pacemaker in this group of patients; which ironically are those that are most likely to benefit. In our experience, patients with documented prolonged asystole associated with vasovagal syncope often benefit from pacemaker implantation.

Hypertrophic obstructive cardiomyopathy has also been a disease process for which pacemaker implantation has been proposed. Early trials showed that pacemaker implantation was beneficial in patients with significant outflow tract gradients.[20–22] The improvement in symptoms was thought to be secondary to an altered sequence of ventricular activation during ventricular pacing leading to a reduction in the outflow tract gradient. However, more recent blinded randomized trials have shown no difference in subjective or objective measures of symptoms or exercise capacity, though patients ≥ 65 years of age appeared to derive symptomatic and functional benefit from pacing in one study.[23,24] As a result of varied responses to pacemaker implantation, most experts agree that pacemaker implantation in patients with hypertrophic cardiomyopathy should be reserved for those who are not candidates for other treatment options (medication, alcohol septal ablation, or surgery). According to the ACC/AHA/NASPE 2002 guidelines, pacemaker implantation is listed as a Class IIb (usefulness/efficacy is less well established by evidence/opinion) indication for patients with hypertrophic cardiomyopathy and symptoms.[2,3]

Summary

The last few decades have witnessed a large growth in the sophistication of current generation pacemakers. Today's pacemakers have moved closer to becoming more physiologic with the ability to sense, pace, modulate rate based on patient activity, pace from multiple sites within one chamber and pace only "as needed." In addition, they also have features to record histograms of heart rate trends as well as arrhythmias, including intracardiac electrograms thereby serving not only a therapeutic function, but also a diagnostic purpose as well. Current indications for pacemakers have expanded to include patients with a variety of indications as the technique for implantation has become easier. In the future, pacemakers will also last longer as further refinements are made in algorithms that enable them to deliver the smallest amount of energy possible while still pacing the heart. As the population ages, all the refinements in pacemaker technology will allow us to be better equipped in treating patients who need to undergo pacemaker implantation.

References

1 Gregoratos G, Abrams J, Epstein AE *et al.* ACC/AHA/NASPE 2002 guideline update for implantation of cardiac pacemakers and antiarrhythmia devices – summary article: a report of the American College of Cardiology/American Heart Association Task Force on Practice Guidelines (ACC/AHA/NASPE Committee to update the 1998 pacemaker guidelines). *J Cardiovasc Electrophysiol* 2002; 13: 1183–99.
2 Gregoratos G, Abrams J, Epstein AE *et al.* ACC/AHA/NASPE 2002 guideline update for implantation of cardiac pacemakers and antiarrhythmia devices – summary article: a report of the American College of Cardiology/American Heart Association Task Force on Practice Guidelines (ACC/AHA/NASPE Committee to update the 1998 pacemaker guidelines). *J Am Coll Cardiol* 2002; 40: 1703–19.

3 Gregoratos G, Abrams J, Epstein AE *et al.* ACC/AHA/NASPE 2002 guideline update for implantation of cardiac pacemakers and antiarrhythmia devices – summary article: a report of the American College of Cardiology/American Heart Association Task Force on Practice Guidelines (ACC/AHA/NASPE Committee to update the 1998 pacemaker guidelines). *Circulation* 2002; 106: 2145–61.

4 Reicin G, Wittes J, Lee W. Notes from Our 7th Annual CRM Conference. Morgan Stanely Hospital Supplies and Medical Technology. September 15, 2003.

5 Kusumoto FM, Goldschlager N. Cardiac pacing. *N Engl J Med* 1996; 334: 89–97.

6 Buckingham TA, Volgman AS, Wimer E. Trends in pacemaker use: results of a multicenter registry. *Pacing Clin Electrophysiol* 1991; 14: 1437–9.

7 Bernstein AD, Daubert JC, Fletcher RD *et al.* The revised NASPE/BPEG generic code for antibradycardia, adaptive-rate, and multisite pacing. North American Society of Pacing and Electrophysiology/British Pacing and Electrophysiology Group. *Pacing Clin Electrophysiol* 2002; 25: 260–4.

8 Sutton R, Kenny RA. The natural history of sick sinus syndrome. *Pacing Clin Electrophysiol* 1986; 9: 1110–4.

9 Wilkoff BL, Cook JR, Epstein AE *et al.* Dual-chamber pacing or ventricular backup pacing in patients with an implantable defibrillator: the Dual Chamber and VVI Implantable Defibrillator (DAVID) Trial. *JAMA* 2002; 288: 3115–23.

10 Lamas GA, Lee KL, Sweeney MO *et al.* Mode Selection Trial in sinus-node dysfunction. Ventricular pacing or dual-chamber pacing for sinus-node dysfunction. *N Engl J Med* 2002; 346: 1854–62.

11 Sweeney MO, Hellkamp AS, Ellenbogen KA *et al.* Adverse effect of ventricular pacing on heart failure and atrial fibrillation among patients with normal baseline QRS duration in a clinical trial of pacemaker therapy for sinus node dysfunction. *Circulation* 2003; 107: 2932–7.

12 Lamas GA, Orav EJ, Stambler BS *et al.* Quality of life and clinical outcomes in elderly patients treated with ventricular pacing as compared with dual-chamber pacing. Pacemaker Selection in the Elderly Investigators. *N Engl J Med* 1998; 338: 1097–104.

13 Toff WD, Skene AM, Camm AJ *et al.* A Prospective comparison of the clinical benefits of dual-chamber versus single chamber ventricular pacing in elderly patients with high-grade atrioventricular block: the United Kingdom Pacing and Cardiovascular Events (UKPACE) Trial [abstract]. *J Am Coll Cardiol* 2003; 41.

14 Sweeney MO, Shea J, Fox V *et al.* Randomized trial of a new minimal ventricular pacing mode in patients with dual chamber ICDs [abstract]. *Pacing Clin Electrophysiol* 2003; 26: 973.

15 Sweeney MO, Shea J, Fox V *et al.* Long AV intervals permit reduction of ventricular pacing in a randomized clinical trial of a new minimal ventricular pacing mode (MVP) in patients with dual chamber ICDs [abstract]. *Pacing Clin Electrophysiol* 2003; 26: 1058.

16 Connolly SJ, Sheldon R, Roberts RS *et al.* The North American Vasovagal Pacemaker Study (VPS). A randomized trial of permanent cardiac pacing for the prevention of vasovagal syncope. *J Am Coll Cardiol* 1999; 33: 16–20.

17 Sutton R, Brignole M, Menozzi C *et al.* Dual-chamber pacing in the treatment of neurally mediated tilt-positive cardioinhibitory syncope: pacemaker versus no therapy: a multicenter randomized study. The Vasovagal Syncope International Study (VASIS) Investigators. *Circulation* 2000; 102: 294–9.

18 Ammirati F, Colivicchi F, Santini M *et al.* Permanent cardiac pacing versus medical treatment for the prevention of recurrent vasovagal syncope: a multicenter, randomized, controlled trial. *Circulation* 2001; 104: 52–7.

19 Connolly SJ, Sheldon R, Thorpe KE *et al.* Pacemaker therapy for prevention of syncope in patients with recurrent severe vasovagal syncope: Second Vasovagal Pacemaker Study (VPS II): a randomized trial. *JAMA* 2003; 289: 2224–9.

20 Jeanrenaud X, Goy JJ, Kappenberger L. Effects of dual-chamber pacing in hypertrophic obstructive cardiomyopathy. *Lancet* 1992; 339: 1318–23.

21 Slade AK, Sadoul N, Shapiro L *et al.* DDD pacing in hypertrophic cardiomyopathy: a multicentre clinical experience. *Heart* 1996; 75: 44–9.

22 Fananapazir L, Epstein ND, Curiel RV *et al.* Long-term results of dual-chamber (DDD) pacing in obstructive hypertrophic cardiomyopathy. Evidence for progressive symptomatic and hemodynamic improvement and reduction of left ventricular hypertrophy. *Circulation* 1994; 90: 2731–42.

23 Nishimura RA, Trusty JM, Hayes DL *et al.* Dual-chamber pacing for hypertrophic cardiomyopathy: a randomized, double-blind, crossover trial. *J Am Coll Cardiol* 1997; 29: 435–41.

24 Maron BJ, Nishimura RA, McKenna WJ *et al.* Assessment of permanent dual-chamber pacing as a treatment for drug-refractory symptomatic patients with obstructive hypertrophic cardiomyopathy. A randomized, double-blind, crossover study (M-PATHY). *Circulation* 1999; 99: 2927–33.

CHAPTER 4

The ICD and how it works

Henry F. Clemo and Kenneth A. Ellenbogen

Introduction

Sudden cardiac death is a national public health problem and it is responsible for over 500 000 deaths per year in the United States alone. The majority of sudden deaths are due to cardiac dysrhythmias, in particular ventricular tachycardia (VT) and ventricular fibrillation (VF). Over the past 25 years, the implantable cardioverter-defibrillator (ICD) has developed to become a device that is now as easily implanted as a pacemaker and can rapidly and successfully resuscitate >99% of patients who develop ventricular tachyarrhythmias. The indications for ICD placement continue to widen and the number of ICDs implanted will only continue to increase in the future.[1]

History of the implantable cardioverter-defibrillator

The concept of defibrillating the heart to convert ventricular tachyarrhythmias to sinus rhythm was brought to reality by Dr P.M. Zoll during the 1940s. Initial work focused on direct defibrillation of the heart in the operating room; later refinements led to the closed chest, transcutaneous defibrillator.[2] Now, the external defibrillator is completely automatic and can be used even by a 12-year-old child. The American Heart Association advocates widespread deployment of automatic external defibrillators (AEDs) in public places.

Dr Michel Mirowski is credited for the development of the ICD. His idea for the ICD arose from seeing his chief of medicine pass out repeatedly from episodes of ventricular tachyarrhythmias. Based on the concept that direct internal defibrillation could successfully defibrillate a patient using 10-fold less energy (30 J versus 300 J) than conventional external defibrillators, Mirowski and his collaborator Morton Mower developed a transvenous right ventricular (RV) defibrillation lead and a left ventricular epicardial patch connected to a generator utilizing off-the-shelf photographic flash capacitors, batteries, switches, and a "home-brew" circuit board. Such a system was initially built, tested, and refined while Dr Mirowski was at the Sinai Hospital in Baltimore

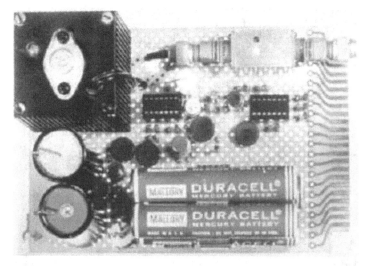

Figure 4.1 Morowski and Mower's first ICD. The first ICD was built with off-the-shelf photographic flash unit capacitors (cylinders at lower left), mercury batteries (lower right), heavy duty switches to allow for charging and discharge of the capacitors (black box at upper left), and crude circuitry to allow for determination of ventricular fibrillation (upper right).

in the late 1960s to the mid 1970s. Their first ICD is shown in Figure 4.1. After the publication of initial results in animals, Dr Bernard Lown, a prominent cardiologist, who developed the concept of the modern coronary care unit, noted that "the implanted defibrillator system represents an imperfect solution in search of a plausible and practical application.[3]"

The first ICD implant in humans took place at Johns Hopkins in 1980. Since that time, critical developments have occurred to transform the ICD from a nonprogrammable device with a weight of 293 g and a volume of 162 mL, which necessitated abdominal implant to a device with a weight of <80 g and size <35 mL that is also programmable, transvenously implanted and capable of delivery of multiple different tiered therapies. An example of a recent defibrillation system that combines atrial and biventricular bradycardia pacing is shown in Figure 4.2. Outlined below are the components of the ICD and how they have developed since Dr Mirowksi's first device.

The basic components of an ICD system consist of leads that are required for sensing the cardiac rhythm and a hermetically sealed can that contains circuitry for analyzing the sensed cardiac electrograms and characterizing the rhythm as supraventricular rhythm, VT, VF, or others. Other components included in the ICD "can" are a battery to supply the necessary energy for sensing, rhythm analysis, and energy delivery to the heart and capacitors for storing the energy prior to shock delivery.

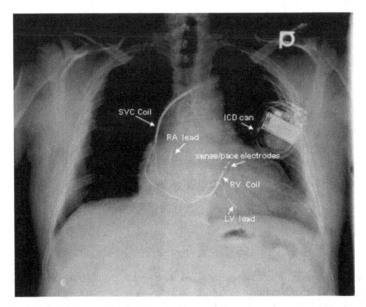

Figure 4.2 Chest radiograph depicting a biventricular or cardiac resynchronization device consisting of biventricular pacing, ventricular defibrillation and atrial and left ventricular leads. Right atrial (RA) lead is positioned in the right atrial appendage (RAA), RV pacing/defibrillation is actively fixed at the right ventricular outflow tract (RVOT) in this example (though it is usually positioned at the RVA), and left ventricular leads have been placed via the left axillary vein and course through the superior vena cava to the right atrium, right ventricle, and coronary sinus to a lateral cardiac vein, respectively. The defibrillation coils on the RV lead can be clearly identified on the X-ray. The ICD can is positioned in a subcutaneous position over the left thorax. ICD = implantable cardioverter-defibrillator, LV = left ventricle, RA = right atrium, RV = right ventricle, SVC = superior vena cava.

ICD leads

Initial ICD leads were epicardially based, with two large patch defibrillation electrodes and two rate sensing electrodes. These leads could only be placed via open chest surgery, with a significant peri- and postoperative morbidity and mortality. The epicardial-rate-sensing leads were associated with a high rate of failure, necessitating frequent revision.

Over the past 15 years, manufacturers have developed a single transvenous lead that incorporates defibrillation electrodes in the right atrium and ventricle, and distal rate-sensing electrodes (Figure 4.3). Defibrillation leads are now not much bigger than a conventional pacing lead (7–9 French) and are easily placed transvenously via the cephalic, axillary, or subclavian vein, thus obviating the need for open chest surgery. Presently, manufacturers are reducing the size of ICD leads as well as increasing the surface area of defibrillation electrodes, which improves defibrillation efficiency.

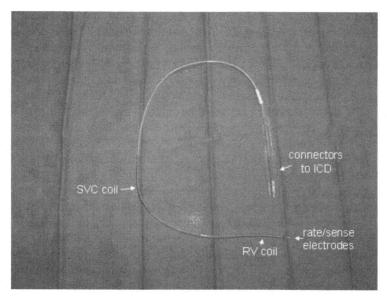

Figure 4.3 RV defibrillation lead. Note the proximal SVC and RV defibrillation coils. The tip of the lead contains a bipolar pace/sense electrode system. The lead is attached via connectors, which plug into a header on the ICD.

While the development of easily placed transvenous defibrillation leads has revolutionized ICD implantation, they often must be removed and replaced, which carries a significant morbidity and mortality. Lead failure due to insulation breakdown or conductor fracture and lead infection both necessitate lead removal. To ease lead removal, laser lead removal systems and also special Gore™ coatings placed over the lead coils have been developed.

ICD lead integrity may be ascertained by determining resistances of the pace/sense and defibrillation electrodes/conductors, the size and quality of recorded intracardiac electrograms, and pacing thresholds. Additionally, electrograms stored by the ICD may indicate noise, possibly caused by conductor or insulation failure. All of this information should be obtained at the time of each ICD device follow-up visit.

ICD generators

The ICD generator is comprised of a battery, capacitors, switches, computer circuitry (processors, memory), telemetry capability, and connectors all contained in a titanium can. The core components, while significantly refined, are similar to those of Mirowski's first ICD (Figure 4.1). Developments in each of these components has led to a 10-fold reduction in size, which now allows the generator to be placed subcutaneously in the pectoral region, much like a pacemaker.

ICD batteries must be capable of high energy storage and a relatively stable voltage output over their lifespan. The batteries are lithium/silver/vanadium, capable of delivering 3.2 V at the beginning of their life. Voltage does gradually decrease over the life of the battery and contributes to progressively longer capacitor charge times. Newer battery chemistries have minimized this decrease in voltage. Future battery developments will include higher energy storage and delivery. Battery status is determined by a combination of measured battery voltage and time to charge the defibrillator capacitor to a set energy, which are obtained each time the device is interrogated. This information allows for determination of elective replacement indicator (ERI) status and timely replacement of the device.

A typical battery by itself cannot deliver enough instantaneous energy to successfully defibrillate a heart. To achieve appropriate energies to defibrillate, ICDs use capacitors that are charged over 3–10 seconds by the ICD battery and then release this energy rapidly for defibrillation. Initial capacitors were cylindrical, bulky, and not designed with ICD generators in mind. Recently, new capacitors that are flat and may be manufactured into a multitude of shapes have been developed to decrease the size of the ICD. The waveform of the capacitor discharge may be monophasic with a single polarity discharge, or biphasic where discharge polarity is divided into two phases of opposite polarity. Biphasic discharge has dramatically improved defibrillation efficiency compared to monophasic discharge, and all current ICDs deliver a biphasic waveform.

In order to function appropriately, the ICD must be able to reliably detect ventricular tachyarrhythmias and then deliver therapy to restore a stable rhythm. The first ICDs had crude circuitry with discrete components with attendant large size and considerable current drain. These defibrillators were not programmable and could only deliver high-energy shocks. Later defibrillators, with downsized electronic components utilizing the new integrated circuit technologies, allowed multiprogrammability of the tachycardia detection rate and also the energy of the delivered shock. Now, ICDs are fully programmable so that different types of therapies based on ventricular rate may be programmed (tiered therapy). These therapies include antitachycardia pacing, low-energy cardioversion, and high-energy cardioversion, depending on the rate of the VT. Additionally, the electrophysiologist may program a variety of supraventricular tachycardia discriminators and bradycardia therapies as well as retrieve a wealth of diagnostic information including lead resistance, pacing and sensing thresholds, and stored intracardiac electrograms immediately before, during, and after delivered therapy.

Ventricular tachyarrhythmia detection

In order to deliver therapy, the ICD must reliably detect the arrhythmia. Initial ICDs used a probability density function algorithm to determine the amount of time the recorded ventricular signal deviated from the baseline. This was based on the assumption that in ventricular fibrillation, the recorded signal was far more likely to deviate from baseline as a function of time than in sinus rhythm. This algorithm proved to be unreliable. Current ICDs use an algorithm based on the rate detected by the ventricular sensing lead to determine when to deliver therapy.

More precisely, the ICD counts ventricular events as a function of time by interpreting signals delivered by the rate-sensing portion of the ICD lead. The sensed signal is filtered with a bandpass filter to remove nonphysiological events. The sensed signal may vary from 0.2 mV in VF to 10 mV or more in sinus rhythm. Appropriate sensing may be disturbed in patients with external or temporary pacemakers, or in the presence of separate implanted pacemakers (not incorporated into the ICD). In addition, low amplitude of sensed signals during VF could result in absence of a sensed signal, leading to delivery of pacing (because the bradycardia pacing components of the ICD "thinks" pacing is required). In such cases, pacemaker spikes (which are not inhibited because of failure to sense VF or VT) can saturate sensing amplifiers resulting in undersensing of VF. Most ICDs now have autogain and autothreshold sensing functions to allow for reliable counting of discrete ventricular events.

The ICD measures the time interval between sensed consecutive ventricular signals and compares this interval to a programmed time interval (i.e. 330 ms or 180 bpm). If a fraction of intervals (e.g. $\frac{2}{3}$ or 12 out of 18) is less than the programmed interval, the ICD interprets this as a ventricular tachyarrhythmia and will deliver therapy. Several detection zones may be programmed, including a VF zone (e.g. interval length less than 300 ms) corresponding to a rate >200 bpm and a VT zone (e.g. intervals falling between 400 ms and 300 ms) corresponding to rates between 150 and 200 bpm. Discrimination between VT and VF allows for therapies to be tailored to each condition. An example of recorded intracardiac electrograms showing VT with a rate of about 240 bpm is shown in Figure 4.4. To satisfy detection of VF, 75% of the ventricular intervals in a "rolling window" (e.g. 18 of 24 cycles) must be less than the programmed cutoff. For VT, a consecutive number of ventricular intervals in a "rolling" window (i.e. 16) must be less than the cutoff rate programmed. A flow diagram of a typical VT and VF detection scheme is shown in Figure 4.5.

Supraventricular tachycardia discrimination

Unfortunately, many supraventricular tachycardias (SVT) such as atrial fibrillation and sinus tachycardia can cause ventricular rates in excess of 150 bpm and potential triggering of inappropriate ventricular tachyarrhythmia therapies. Early ICDs had a >25% inappropriate therapy rate.[4] Since that time, ventricular arrhythmia detection enhancements have evolved to reduce the potential to inappropriately detect SVT.

In single chamber ICDs (systems without an atrial lead), detection enhancements include rapidity of onset, rate stability, and intrinsic QRS morphology.

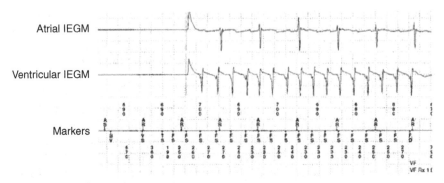

Figure 4.4 Example of a stored intracardiac electrogram (IEGM) retrieved from the memory of a defibrillator. The top tracing shows the sensed atrial IEGM, and the middle the ventricular IEGM. The bottom tracing labeled "Markers" depicts time intervals (in ms) between atrial events (labeled AR) and between ventricular events (labeled BV–biventricular pacing, TS–VT sensing, and FS VF sensing). Note that the first beat (IEGMs not shown) is sensing in the atrium followed by a paced beat (AS-BV). Next is a ventricular sensed event, which is probably a premature ventricular contraction (PVC) followed by an atrial escape beat (VS-AR). The next ventricular beat occurs 360 ms later (labeled TS given the interval time). The ventricular rate accelerates to an interval length of 230–270 ms, which falls in the VF zone (labeled FS). There are 18 consecutive FS beats, which satisfies an 18 of 24 beat criteria to be labeled a VF event (denoted FD, fibrillation detect). Note that there is ventriculo atrial dissociation with an atrial escape interval of 680–700 ms, much longer than the VF interval.

These enhancements are described further in Table 4.1. All of the SVT criteria that are programmed "on" must be met to suppress therapy. If any one criterion is not met, the ICD assumes that a ventricular arrhythmia is present and will deliver therapy. All ICDs also have a "sustained high rate duration" parameter (i.e. duration of time during which the rate remains elevated regardless of the SVT discrimination criteria), which when exceeded triggers the ICD to deliver therapy.

The addition of an atrial lead to the ICD system allows incorporation of atrial rhythm data into SVT discrimination algorithms. Additional parameters that may be programmed include atrial rate > ventricular rate and timing of atrial depolarization relative to ventricular depolarization. These parameters can help differentiate rapid-onset SVTs from VT. The addition of atrial data to SVT algorithms has reduced inappropriate detections to about 10–20%.

Tachyarrhythmia therapies

VT at rates of up to 200 bpm can be converted to baseline rhythm with a >80% efficacy using overdrive-pacing algorithms (antitachycardia pacing, or "ATP"). This is painless to the patient and minimizes ICD battery drain. Once VT is

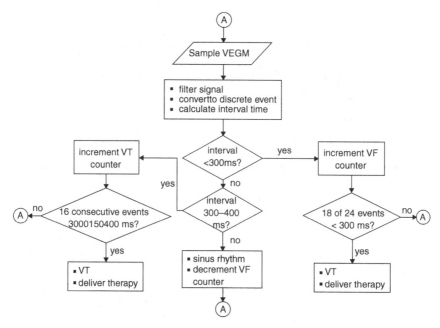

Figure 4.5 Algorithm for VT and VF detection. At point A, the ICD samples the ventricular electrogram (VEGM) and calculates an interval between discrete ventricular events. Decision making based on yes/no criteria is then made to classify whether the interval falls in a VT or VF zone. If the interval meets criteria for either VT or VF, counters are incremented. When a certain number of intervals meet rate criteria, therapy is then delivered.

Table 4.1 SVT detection enhancements

Parameter	Utility	Pitfalls
Onset	Detects slowly accelerating SVT such as ST	AFIB or AFL are rapid in onset
Stability	Detects irregular rates seen in AFIB	Reentrant SVTs often have stable ventricular response
QRS morphology	VT QRS different than SVT	Subtle changes in QRS related to rate can confound QRS morphology

Note: AFIB – atrial fibrillation; AFL – atrial flutter.

detected, if ATP therapy is programmed on, pacing therapy will be delivered. Typically, several attempts at overdrive pacing will be programmed as initial therapy for VT. After each therapy delivery, the ICD checks for conversion to sinus rhythm or continuation of VT or acceleration of VT. Subsequent therapies are based on the continuing VT rate. In about 5% of cases, overdrive pacing may accelerate VT to VF, which would then precipitate a high-energy

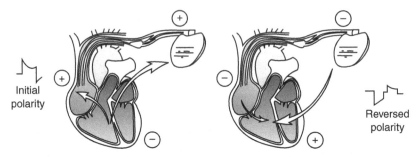

Figure 4.6 Demonstration of shock polarity in a transvenous ICD system. Capacitor discharge waveform is shown to the left and the right (reversed initial polarity) of the figure. Shocks are delivered from the RV coil to the SVC coil/ICD can. The ICD can is termed "active."

defibrillation shock from the device.[5] Once overdrive-pacing attempts are exhausted, the ICD then will attempt low-energy cardioversion followed by high-energy defibrillation.

The ICD delivers shocks via discharge from capacitors, which are charged by a battery. Capacitor discharge follows an exponential decay, which is influenced by the capacitor characteristics and resistance of the electrode system. Most ICDs release 60% or more of the total energy stored in the charged capacitors in less than 20 ms. As mentioned above, the polarity is reversed toward the end of discharge to make the discharge waveform biphasic. This improves defibrillation efficiency dramatically. Two capacitors are typically used in series and are capable of delivering energy of about 27–34 J. The amplitude of energy may be programmed, since low energy cardioversions are quite efficacious at converting VT to sinus rhythm and also require shorter capacitor charge times. Energy delivery is delivered between the metal can of the ICD combined with the SVC coil to the RV electrode, as demonstrated in Figure 4.6. Prior to shock delivery, typically after capacitor charging, the device will "reconfirm" that VF or VT is still present before the shock is delivered.

A defibrillation threshold (DFT) is determined at time of device implant. The DFT is defined as the lowest amount of energy required to reliably convert VF to the baseline rhythm. In most patients, the DFT is less than 20 J, which allows for a >10 J safety margin for the typical ICD, which is capable of delivering 30 J per shock. When a suitable DFT cannot be obtained, revision of the ICD system including lead repositioning, insertion of additional leads placed transvenously or subcutaneously, or substitution of a high-energy output ICD may be needed.

Bradyarrhythmia pacing therapies

Many patients, who receive ICDs, also have sinus node or conduction system disease, putting them at risk for bradyarrhythmias. These patients may require pacing for prevention of bradycardia. ICDs, which incorporate both atrial and ventricular leads, are capable of dual chamber rate adaptive (DDDR) pacing. Unfortunately, excessive pacing from the right ventricular apex (RVA) in the ICD patient may lead to an increased incidence of congestive heart failure and atrial fibrillation. Some patients may have evidence of left ventricular dyssynchrony and may benefit from cardiac resynchronization with the addition of a left ventricular lead, which is placed from the right atrium via the coronary sinus and into a lateral cardiac vein. An example of a biventricular ICD is shown in Figure 4.2.

The future

The indications for ICD implantation are rapidly expanding as a result of recent clinical trials demonstrating mortality reduction with ICD therapy in post-myocardial infarction and congestive heart failure patients. This will have a profound effect on health-care costs. ICD manufacturers are thus under pressure to produce a low cost, easy to implant systems. ICD and lead technology will continue to improve, but it is unlikely that the size of devices will significantly reduce further, restricted by the limitations of current capacitor technology and the energy required to defibrillate the heart.

It may also be feasible to develop an entirely subcutaneous defibrillation leads for the ICD in the future, though such a system may have limited diagnostic features and would be unable to provide overdrive or bradycardia pacing. A further potential area of improvement in the ICD is the incorporation of diagnostic and therapeutic features for management of congestive heart failure. New devices currently undergoing clinical trials can determine pulmonary resistance, which may be used as a guide for heart failure therapies.

References

1 The Antiarrhythmic Versus Implantable Defibrillator (AVID) Investigators. A comparison of antiarrhythmic-drug therapy with implantable defibrillators in patients resuscitated from near-fatal ventricular arrhythmias. *N Engl J Med* 1997; 337: 1576–83.

2 Buxton AE, Lee DL, Fisher JD *et al*. A randomized study of the prevention of sudden death in patients with coronary artery disease. *N Engl J Med* 1999; 341: 1882–90.

3 Ellenbogen KA, Kay GN, Wilkoff BL (eds). *Clinical Cardiac Pacing and Defibrillation*. Philadelphia: W.B. Saunders, 2000.

4 The DAVID investigators. Dual chamber pacing or ventricular backup pacing in patients with an implantable defibirillator. *JAMA* 2002; 288: 3115–23.

5 Epstein AE, Miles WM, Benditt DG *et al*. Personal and public safety issues related to arrhythmias that may affect consciousness: implications for regulation and physician recommendations. A medical/scientific statement from the American heart Association and the North American Society of Pacing and Electrophysiology. *Circulation* 1996; 94: 1147–66.

6 Gregoratos G, Abrans J, Epstein AE *et al.* ACC/AHA/NASPE 2002 guideline update for implantation of cardiac pacemakers and antiarrhythmia devices: a report of the American College or Cardiology/American Heart Association Task Force on Practice Guidelines (ACC/AHA/NASPE Committee on Pacemaker Implantation). *J Am Coll Cardiol* 2002; 40: 1703–19.

7 Zoll PM, Linenthal AJ, Gibson W, Paul MH and Norman LR. Termination of ventricular fibrillation in man by externally applied countershock, *N Engl J Med* 1956; 254: 727–32.

8 Lown B, Axelrod P. Implanted standby defibrillators. *Circulation* 1972; 46: 637–9.

9 Nisam S. Technology update: the modern implantable cardioverter defibrillator. *Ann Noninvasive Electrocardiol* 1997; 2: 69–78.

10 Schaumann A, Von zur Mühlen F, Herse B *et al.* Empirical versus tested antitachycardia pacing in implantable cardioverter defibrillators: A prospective study including 200 patients. *Circulation* 1998; 97: 66–74.

11 Kaul Y, Mohan JC, Gopinath N *et al.* Permanent pacemaker infections: their characterization and management: a 15-year experience. *Indian Heart J* 1983; 35: 345–9.

12 Kühlkamp K, Dörnberger V, Mewis C *et al.* Clinical experience with the new detection algorithms for atrial fibrillation of a defibrillator with dual chamber sensing and pacing. *J Cardiovasc Electrophysiol* 1999; 10: 905–15.

13 Mela T, McGovern BA, Garan H *et al.* Long-term infection rates associated with the pectoral versus abdominal approach to cardioverter-defibrillator implants. *Am J Cardiol* 2001; 88: 750–3.

14 Moss A, Hall J, Cannom D *et al.* Improved survival with an implanted defibrillator in patients with coronary disease at high risk ventricular arrhythmias. *N Engl J Med* 1997; 335: 1933–40.

15 Moss AJ, Zareba W, Hall WJ *et al.* Prophylactic implantation of a defibrillator in patients with myocardial infarction and reduced ejection fraction. *N Engl J Med* 2002; 346: 877–83.

CHAPTER 5
Indications for the implanted cardioverter-defibrillator

Alfred E. Buxton

The implantable defibrillator was introduced to clinical medicine in 1980.[1] This device, invented by Michel Mirowski, has revolutionized the care of patients with ventricular arrhythmias. Spurred by an array of technical refinements and a multitude of clinical trials documenting efficacy, the use of the implantable cardioverter-defibrillator (ICD) has grown exponentially.[2] About 10–15 years ago, initial treatment of most ventricular arrhythmias was antiarrhythmic drugs. In the United States, it is no longer thought that the ICD should be used only after a test or clinical event to suggest drug failure. This change has resulted from increasing realization of both the hazards and the limited efficacy of current pharmacologic antiarrhythmic agents. In addition, multiple randomized clinical trials have demonstrated improved survival of patients treated with the ICD in comparison with pharmacologic therapy. There is no doubt that the ICD effectively terminates most episodes of ventricular fibrillation (VF) by a shock, and ventricular tachycardia (VT) by pacing or shock. However, the cost of this technology is significant. At the same time that increasing numbers of clinical trials have demonstrated utility of the ICD, there are few data to determine the optimal way in which to risk-stratify patients who may be at risk, but have yet to experience a spontaneous episode of sustained VT or VF. Indications for ICDs are evolving continuously. This chapter reviews current ICD indications and the data that form the basis for them. Readers should be aware that as this chapter is being written, an update of guidelines recommended by the joint American College of Cardiology/American Heart Association/European Society of Cardiology Committee on Ventricular Arrhythmias and Sudden Cardiac Death is in preparation. In this chapter, the rationale (clinical trial data) supporting the current consensus recommendations of the European Society of Cardiology, the American Heart Association, and the American College of Cardiology has been reviewed.

Primary versus secondary prevention of sudden cardiac death

There are two major indications for use of the ICD: primary and secondary prevention of sudden cardiac death. Primary prevention refers to the prophylactic use of an ICD in patients who have characteristics that identify them as being at high risk for sudden death, but have never experienced a symptomatic sustained tachycardia. Secondary prevention refers to the treatment of patients who have survived a cardiac arrest or an episode of sustained VT that has resulted in severe hemodynamic compromise. Emerging data suggest that ICDs can be useful to prevent sudden death in patients at risk due to a variety of conditions but who have never experienced a symptomatic arrhythmia, though the indications are not as well established as those for survivors of cardiac arrest.

Summary of ICD recommendations: secondary prevention

1 The primary therapy for survivors of cardiac arrest or sustained VT resulting in severe hemodynamic compromise is the ICD, after reversible causes are corrected.
2 The ICD is an effective therapy for patients with symptomatic sustained monomorphic VT that does not cause significant hemodynamic compromise.

Basis for recommendations

Patients experiencing cardiac arrest due to VT or VF that does not occur within the first 24 hours of an acute myocardial infarction (AMI) are at high risk for recurrent arrest or sudden death. Clinical studies have demonstrated event rates of 25–30% over 1–2 years follow-up.[3] Such patients should be evaluated and treated for myocardial ischemia. If there is a clear evidence that acute ischemia immediately preceded the onset of the ventricular tachyarrhythmia, if systolic ventricular function is within normal limits [usually measured by ejection fraction (EF)], and there is no evidence of prior infarction, the primary therapy should be coronary revascularization. However, if revascularization cannot be performed, or there is evidence of prior MI, or significant left ventricular (LV) dysfunction after recovery from the acute event, the primary therapy of patients resuscitated from cardiac arrest due to VT or VF should be the ICD. It is important to recognize that when LV function is evaluated shortly after a cardiac arrest, the EF will usually be depressed. The LV function often recovers to normal levels in patients without preexisting systolic ventricular dysfunction that do not evolve a new MI at the time of the arrest. Thus, evaluation of ventricular function should probably be delayed 1–2 weeks after cardiac arrest.

This ICD recommendation stems from the results of several large-scale randomized trials comparing outcome of cardiac arrest survivors treated with ICDs versus drugs (Tables 5.1–5.3). The largest of these trials, the Antiarrhythmics Versus Implantable Defibrillators Trial (AVID),[4] studied 1016 patients (Tables 5.1 and 5.2). Patients were randomized to therapy with ICD or an antiarrhythmic drug. The drug therapy choices were empiric amiodarone,

Table 5.1 Secondary prevention trials – enrollment criteria

Trial	Spontaneous arrhythmia or event	Treatment
AVID[4]	Near fatal VF	Antiarrhythmic drugs (amiodarone or sotalol)
	Sustained VT with syncope	ICD
	Sustained VT, EF $\leq$ 0.40, and symptoms suggesting severe hemodynamic compromise	
CASH[5]	Cardiac arrest secondary to documented sustained ventricular arrhythmias	Antiarrhythmic drugs (amiodarone, metoprolol, propafenone*) ICD
	Documented VF	Amiodarone
	Out-of-hospital cardiac arrest requiring defibrillation of cardioversion	ICD
	Documeneted sustained VT causing syncope	
	Other documented, sustained VT, rate $\geq$150 bpm causing presyncope or angina in patient with EF $\leq$ 0.35	
	Unmonitored syncope with subsequent documentation of either spontaneous VT lasting at least 10 s. Or sustained monomorphic VT induced by EP	

Notes: AVID – Antiarrhythmics Versus Implantable Defibrillators Trial. CASH – Cardiac Arrest Survivors Hamburg Trial. CIDS – Canadian Implantable Defibrillator Study. VF – ventricular fibrillation. VT – ventricular tachycardia. ICD – implantable cardioverter-defibrillator. EP – electrophysiologic study.

*The propafenone treatment arm in CASH was terminated prematurely, after an interim analysis showed 61% higher mortality than ICD-treated patients after follow-up of 11.3 months. Patients randomized to propafenone are not considered in the outcome results.

Table 5.2 Secondary prevention trials – patient characteristics

Trial	N	Age (years, mean)	Gender (% male)	Index arrhythmia VF/VT (%)	CAD (%)	No structural heart disease (%)	EF (%)	HF at enrollment None/Class I,II / III (%)
AVID	1016	65	78, 81	45/55	81	3	32	43 / 48 / 10
CASH	288	58	80	84/16	73	10	46	27 / 56 / 17
CIDS	659	63	85	48/13/25/14*	82	3	34	50 / 39 / 11

Notes: Abbreviations as in Table 5.1. N – number patients randomized. CAD – coronary artery disease. EF – ejection fraction. HF – heart failure. Class refers to NYHA functional class at time of enrollment. Values shown refer to mean values for all enrolled patients in each study.

*The distribution of Index Arrhythmias for patients enrolled in CIDS represents patients with: VF or cardiac arrest / VT with syncope / Other VT / Unmonitored syncope, respectively.

Table 5.3 Secondary prevention trials – results

Trial	Follow-up, months (mean)	2-year survival control group (%)	2-year survival ICD group (%)	Mortality reduction associated with ICD therapy (%)
AVID	18.2	74.7	81.6	38
CASH	57	80.4*	88	24
CIDS	36	79.03	85.25	18

Notes: Abbreviations as in Table 5.1.
*Survival figures for CASH control group refer to patients randomized to amiodarone and metoprolol combined.

or sotalol (following either an electrophysiologic test or Holter monitor to predict efficacy). The majority (483 of 509) of patients randomized to receive drug therapy were treated with amiodarone. Patients randomized to ICD therapy demonstrated improved survival compared to those randomized to drug therapy. After a mean follow-up of 18.2 months, 15.8% of patients treated with ICDs had died, compared to 24% of patients randomized to drug therapy. ICD therapy was associated with a relative reduction in total mortality of approximately 30%. The survival benefits associated with ICD therapy in cardiac arrest survivors may not be distributed equally. For example, in patients with higher EFs (e.g. >35%), a substudy of the AVID trial suggested that amiodarone may be equal in efficacy to the ICD.[5] However, it should be remembered that patients with higher EFs seem to have ventricular tachyarrhythmias at a lower frequency than do patients with lower EFs.[6,7] Thus, when a trial such as the AVID study, having a short follow-up duration (18 months average) finds that patients with higher EFs do equally well with the alternative therapies, one must wonder whether the apparent equal efficacy is due merely to the fact that the patients were not observed long enough for potentially lethal recurrent arrhythmias to occur, thereby failing to reveal one therapy as superior to the other.

After publication of the AVID results two other randomized trials of cardiac arrest survivors or severe sustained VT were completed. The Cardiac Arrest Study Hamburg (CASH) randomized 346 survivors of cardiac arrest among four treatment arms: ICD, amiodarone, metoprolol, or propafenone[8] (Tables 5.1 and 5.2). The propafenone arm was terminated prematurely because of excessive mortality (2.6 times that of the ICD arm). After a mean follow-up of 57 months, total mortality was similar for patients randomized to metoprolol and amiodarone (45.4% and 43.5%, respectively). Total mortality of patients randomized to ICD therapy was 35.4%. In comparison to the combined metoprolol and amiodarone patient groups, the ICD-treated patients demonstrated a 23% relative reduction in total mortality ($p = 0.081$).

A third trial, the Canadian Implantable Defibrillator Study (CIDS) randomized 659 survivors of cardiac arrest or hemodynamically unstable VT to therapy

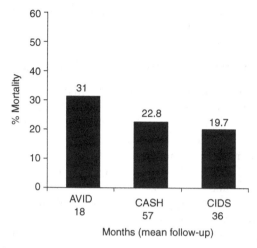

Figure 5.1 Mortality reductions associated with ICD therapy versus antiarrhythmic drugs in secondary prevention trials. Columns depict the reported total mortality reductions for each trial.

with amiodarone or ICD.[9] After a mean follow-up of 3 years, a 20% relative reduction in mortality was observed in patients treated with ICDs compared to that of patients randomized to amiodarone ($p = .142$).

Of these three trials, only the AVID study resulted in a statistically significant reduction in mortality with ICD therapy. However, a formal meta-analysis of the three trials suggested remarkable similarity with respect to patient characteristics and outcome.[10] Overall, therapy with ICDs resulted in a 27% reduction in total mortality and a 51% reduction in arrhythmic mortality. (Figure 5.1). Thus, the ability of ICDs to treat ventricular tachyarrhythmias reduces total mortality as well as the expected risk of arrhythmic deaths.

A number of practical questions relating to patient management are unclear at this time. For example, it is recommended that patients who experience cardiac arrest as a result of transient or reversible causes do not require ICD therapy (assuming that the abnormality is corrected permanently). However, which transient or reversible etiologies constitute an appropriate excuse from the ICD requirement is less than clear. A *post hoc* analysis from the AVID study suggested that patients experiencing cardiac arrest presumed due to transient metabolic perturbations such as hypokalemia or ischemia are at high mortality risk.[11] It is important to recognize that electrolyte abnormalities, such as hypokalemia, often occur secondary to cardiac arrest. As a result, most survivors of cardiac arrest due to VF or polymorphic VT in whom electrolyte abnormalities are discovered should be treated just as survivors of cardiac arrest without electrolyte abnormalities. Likewise, it is important to understand that transient metabolic derangements are rarely the cause of monomorphic sustained VT. Therefore, most patients who experience sustained monomorphic VT that results in significant hemodynamic compromise should be treated with ICDs, regardless of the presence of electrolyte abnormalities.

Ventricular arrhythmias and acute ischemia

Numerous studies have shown that primary VF in the setting of AMI, although associated with increased in-hospital mortality, is not associated with an increased long-term risk of recurrent VF in comparison to patients who do not suffer primary VF.[12–14] Thus, patients who experience primary VF in the acute phase of MI do not require further evaluation or therapy for prevention of sudden death, unless other risk factors are present (*vide infra*). At this time, we do not have data available from controlled trials on the efficacy of myocardial revascularization as sole therapy for patients with polymorphic VT or VF. However, observational studies suggest that sustained monomorphic VT in patients with prior MI is unlikely to be affected by revascularization.[15] Furthermore, myocardial revascularization is unlikely to prevent recurrent cardiac arrest in patients with markedly abnormal LV function, even if the original arrhythmia appeared to result from transient ischemia.[16] Thus, myocardial revascularization is considered adequate as the sole therapy *only* in patients surviving an episode of VF or polymorphic VT in association with myocardial ischemia when ventricular function is normal, and there is no history of MI. Conversely, it is clear that prolonged episodes of sustained monomorphic VT may be associated with a rise in cardiac enzymes such as troponin, due to myocardial metabolic demands outstripping supply. This is a very different problem than that of VF complicating acute infarction described above. Patients with sustained monomorphic VT should be treated similarly, regardless of whether an enzyme rise is documented or not.

Do all patients with VT need an ICD?

The ICD will not necessarily improve the survival of all patients with sustained VT. The three randomized trials comparing ICD to pharmacologic antiarrhythmic therapy did not enroll patients who presented with hemodynamically stable VT. Rather, they required patients who have survived a cardiac arrest or an episode of VT that resulted in severe hemodynamic compromise. The effect of ICD therapy on survival of patients with prior MI and hemodynamically stable sustained monomorphic VT is unclear. These patients may be treated with antiarrhythmic drugs or surgical or radiofrequency catheter ablation, with relatively low risk of sudden death (2–3% yearly).[17,18] Another substudy from the AVID trial registry found high total mortality in patients who presented with hemodynamically stable VT.[19] Of note, the high mortality in the registry occurred in spite of the use of ICDs in 30–40% of such patients. High total mortality in patients who present with sustained VT after MI has been noted previously, and is not surprising, given the significant LV dysfunction present in most such patients.[18] It is important to recognize that although the ICD may not reduce the already low risk of sudden death of patients who present with stable sustained VT after MI, it is a very useful aid in the management of such patients through the use of antitachycardia pacing to terminate tachycardia episodes.

Other patients with sustained monomorphic VT at low risk for sudden death are those with certain types of idiopathic VT in the setting of normal ventricular function. This includes patients with idiopathic VT arising from the right or left ventricular outflow tracts, and "fascicular" LV VT. Such patients, when symptomatic, are best treated by a curative radiofrequency catheter ablation procedure with very high success rates, not the ICD. Finally, it should be recognized that other less common sustained ventricular tachyarrhythmias, such as tachycardia due to bundle branch reentry that may cause syncope or cardiac arrest in patients with cardiomyopathy, are readily cured by radiofrequency catheter ablation.[20] Electrophysiologic testing is required to confirm this mechanism of arrhythmia, which should be considered especially in patients presenting with tachycardia having a left bundle branch block, and left axis configuration.

Other secondary prevention indications

Use of the ICD is now accepted, with a lesser degree of supportive evidence, in several other groups of patients in addition to cardiac arrest survivors. Certain patients with spontaneous sustained VT may be at high risk for sudden death. This includes some patients with VT associated with syncope, or severely symptomatic VT associated with a LV EF <0.40. The AVID trial included 561 patients with sustained VT, and the improvement in survival with ICD therapy observed in these patients was similar to that of patients presenting with VF.

Another group of patients for whom the ICD is accepted as reasonable therapy includes patients with cardiomyopathy who present with syncope of unknown origin, in whom hemodynamically significant sustained VT or VF is induced at electrophysiologic study. This indication is not supported by evidence from randomized clinical trials. Rather, observational data have documented a 20% yearly cardiovascular mortality in such patients, with a large proportion occurring suddenly.[21] Patients with syncope of unclear etiology (after undergoing complete electrophysiologic evaluation) with non-ischemic dilated cardiomyopathy who receive ICDs have a 40–50% incidence of receiving "appropriate" ICD therapies over 2 years.[22,23] This rate of therapy delivery is comparable to that of patients with similar underlying disease who received ICDs as treatment for cardiac arrest. A related indication includes patients with recurrent syncope of uncertain etiology in the presence of severe ventricular dysfunction, who have no inducible ventricular tachyarrhythmias at electrophysiology (EP) study if other causes of syncope are excluded. This group of patients also has a high mortality, with a large proportion occurring suddenly.

Summary of ICD recommendations: primary prevention

The use of ICDs for primary prevention of sudden cardiac death represents a natural evolution of our attempts to reduce mortality of patients with both coronary, as well as noncoronary heart disease. It is based on several lines of evidence. First, sudden unexpected deaths currently account for at least half the mortality of patients with cardiac disease.[24] Second, in most areas of the United States, a minority of persons experiencing out-of-hospital cardiac arrest will survive this event.[25] Thus, prevention of the event is central if we are to significantly reduce mortality from this disease. Third, most victims of cardiac arrest have a known heart disease, and at least in the case of patients with coronary heart disease (responsible for about three-quarters of sudden deaths) a number of clinical parameters have been identified that increase the risk for sudden death. Based upon this knowledge, several large-scale clinical trials have enrolled patients having one or more markers of high mortality risk, and compared survival with ICD therapy versus either empiric pharmacologic anti-arrhythmic therapy, or standard medical therapy alone (nonantiarrhythmic drugs, including β-adrenergic blocking agents and converting enzyme inhibitors). With one exception, these trials were designed to compare the efficacy of ICD versus the alternative therapy to improve survival. Only one trial (the Multicenter UnSustained Tachycardia Trial, or MUSTT) was designed to test a strategy for guiding antiarrhythmic therapy.[26] Thus, most of our current evidence regarding the efficacy of ICDs to reduce mortality of patients with heart disease is based on studies designed to assess ICD efficacy, rather than test the optimal strategy to guide utilization of the ICD.

The primary prevention indications for use of ICDs are less well defined than those for secondary prevention, and are likely to evolve as results from recently completed clinical trials are published. Nonetheless, the joint Guidelines Committee has developed recommendations based on the available evidence.

The major recommendations for primary prevention of sudden death state that:

1 ICD therapy is indicated >40 days after MI in patients with NYHA (New York Heart Association) Class II or III heart failure symptoms whose EF is 30% or less. In the case of patients undergoing coronary artery bypass grafting, implantation should be delayed for 3 or more months after surgery. The EF should be verified at that time after surgery. This recommendation is supported by evidence from multiple randomized controlled trials.[27,28]

2 ICD therapy may be utilized >40 days after MI in patients without symptomatic heart failure when the EF is 30% or less. This recommendation is supported by evidence from one randomized trial.[27]

3 ICD therapy is reasonable >40 days after MI in patients whose EF is between 30% and 40%, who have spontaneous NSVT (nonsustained ventricular tachycardia) and inducible sustained VT.

4 ICD therapy is recommended to reduce the risk of sudden cardiac death in patients with chronic congestive heart failure (due to coronary disease or nonischemic dilated cardiomyopathy), NYHA Functional Class II or III, and LVEF ≤ 30%.

Basis for recommendations

Data from several prospective randomized clinical trials support a role for the ICD in the primary prevention of sudden death, both in patients with coronary heart disease, as well as heart failure due to nonischemic dilated cardiomyopathy. Five of these trials studied patients with coronary artery disease and left ventricular dysfunction, plus or minus other markers of mortality risk (Table 5.1).[27,29–32] Four of the five were designed to specifically evaluate ICD therapy versus a control group [Multicenter Automatic Defibrillator Implantation Trial (MADIT), Coronary Artery Bypass Graft (CABG)-Patch, MADIT II, Defibrillator in Acute Myocardial Infarction Trial (DINAMIT)]. In contrast, the fifth trial, the Multicenter Unsustained Tachycardia Trial (MUSTT), was designed to evaluate a strategy of using electrophysiologic studies to guide antiarrhythmic therapy, pharmacologic as well as ICD (Tables 5.4–5.6).

These studies evaluated patients with coronary artery disease, LV dysfunction, and asymptomatic nonsustained VT. The first of these, the MADIT performed electrophysiologic studies (EPS) in patients with the characteristics noted above.[30] Patients with inducible sustained VT were given intravenous procainamide. If inducible sustained VT persisted, they were then randomized to receive either an ICD or "conventional" antiarrhythmic therapy. The latter

Table 5.4 Primary prevention trials in patients with coronary heart disease – Enrollment Criteria

Trial	Ejection fraction	Spontaneous arrhythmia	Additional entry criteria	Reference
CABG-Patch	≤0.35	None	Abnormal signal-averaged ECG Elective coronary bypass surgery	26,27
MADIT	≤0.35	Nonsustained VT	EP study demonstrating inducible sustained VT not suppressed by procainamide	22
MUSTT	≤0.40	Nonsustained VT	EP study demonstrating inducible sustained VT	21,23,24
MADIT II	≤0.30	None required	None	25,28
DINAMIT	≤0.35	None required	Abnormal HRV or elevated average HR on 24 h monitor	30

Notes: CABG-Patch – Coronary Artery Bypass Graft Patch trial. MADIT – Multicenter Automatic Defibrillator Implantation Trial. MUSTT – Multicenter UnSustained Tachycardia Trial. EP study – Electrophysiologic test utilizing programmed stimulation. DINAMIT – Defibrillator in Acute Myocardial Infarction Trial. HRV – heart rate variability. HR – heart rate.

Table 5.5 Primary prevention trials in patients with coronary heart disease – treatment strategy

	Control group (N)	Active treatment group therapy (N)
CABG-Patch	No antiarrhythmic therapy $N = 454$	ICD placed at time of elective CABG surgery $N = 446$
MADIT	"Conventional" antiarrhythmic drug chosen by investigator (empiric amiodarone in 74%) $N = 101$	ICD $N = 95$
MUSTT	No antiarrhythmic therapy $N = 353$	Antiarrhythmic therapy guided by results of EP testing. If a drug could not be found to prevent inducible VT, patients underwent ICD placement. $N = 351$
MADIT II	No antiarrhythmic therapy $N = 490$	ICD $N = 742$
DINAMIT	No antiarrhythmic therapy $N = 342$	ICD $N = 332$

Notes: Abbreviations as in Table 5.4.

Table 5.6 Primary prevention trials in patients with coronary heart disease – patient characteristics

Trial	Age (years, mean)	Gender (% male)	EF (%)	HF at enrollment NYHA Class II or III (%)	β-blocker Rx control patients (%)	ACE-Inhibitor Rx control patients (%)
CABG-Patch	64	84	27	72	24	53.8
MADIT	63	92	26	65	8	58
MUSTT	67	90	30	63	51	77
MADIT II	64	84	23	59*	70	72
DINAMIT	62	76	28	88	87	94

*In MADIT II an additional 5% of patients were NYHA Class IV.
Percents of β-blocker and ACE-inhibitor therapy represent utilization at enrollment. Percentages were similar for both drug classes for control and ICD treated patients for all trials except MADIT (26% of ICD-treated patients in MADIT received β-blockers).

treatment was uncontrolled, and left to the individual investigators' discretion. Empiric amiodarone was the choice in 74% of cases randomized to this arm. There was no untreated control group in this study. Total mortality was 54% lower for patients randomized to ICD treatment.

The second prospective trial supporting the use of ICDs for primary prevention of sudden death is the MUSTT.[31] The primary aim of this randomized,

Table 5.7 Primary prevention trials in patients with coronary heart disease – results

Trial	Follow-up, months (mean)	2-year survival control group (%)	2-year survival ICD group (%)	Hazard Ratio for ICD therapy (total mortality)
CABG-Patch	32	82	83	1.07
MADIT	27	68	87	0.46
MUSTT	39	72	89	0.45
MADIT II	20	78	84	0.69
DINAMIT	30	85	85	1.08

controlled trial was to assess the ability of antiarrhythmic therapy (including both ICDs and drugs) guided by EPS to reduce the risk of sudden death in patients with coronary artery disease and the other characteristics noted above. Patients who had sustained VT inducible by EPS were randomized into two groups: one received conservative medical therapy, without specific antiarrhythmic treatment while a second group received antiarrhythmic therapy guided by EPS. In the latter group, antiarrhythmic drugs were tested first, and patients who failed to respond to drugs (judged by EPS) then received an ICD. This trial was not designed to compare the efficacy of antiarrhythmic drugs versus the ICD to improve survival. However, at the trial's completion, the number of patients treated with ICDs was approximately the same as those treated with antiarrhythmic drugs in the EP therapy arm. Further analysis demonstrated that the improved survival of the EP-guided group was due entirely to therapy with ICDs.[33] Patients discharged without ICDs had event rates very similar to those of the untreated control patients, while the ICD reduced the risk of arrhythmic death or cardiac arrest by approximately 74% and total mortality was reduced by 50%.[23]

The results of these two trials demonstrated, for the first time, the ability of the ICD to reduce mortality of patients at high risk for sudden death, who had never experienced a symptomatic arrhythmia. The MUSTT trial also established the risk for arrhythmic death or cardiac arrest of patients with coronary disease, LV dysfunction, or asymptomatic nonsustained VT, who have inducible sustained VT. The control group in this trial, treated with β-blocking agents and ACE-inhibitors alone, experienced a Kaplan–Meier 5-year arrhythmic event rate of 32%, and total mortality of 48%. It should be noted that in both the MUSTT and MADIT trials, ICDs were implanted only in patients who failed to respond to antiarrhythmic drugs, as tested in the EP laboratory. Thus, neither trial proved efficacy in patients who respond to drugs at EP testing. However, given the rather poor outcome of patients treated with antiarrhythmic drugs guided by EP testing in the MUSTT trial, it does not seem reasonable to require drug failure prior to ICD use in appropriate patients.

The third primary prevention trial in patients with coronary disease was the MADIT-II study.[27] This trial enrolled patients who experienced a MI at least 1 month previously, had an EF ≤30%, and no symptomatic arrhythmia.

No further risk stratification was performed. Patients were randomized to receive conventional medical therapy or an ICD plus standard therapy. After a mean follow-up period of only 20 months, patients randomized to ICD therapy experienced 31% lower mortality (total mortality 19.8% in the control group, 14.2% in the ICD treated group).

Two primary prevention trials in patients with coronary disease failed to demonstrate any survival benefit with ICD therapy – the CABG-Patch and the DINAMIT trials.[29,32] CABG-Patch tested the hypothesis that ICDs can reduce mortality when implanted in patients undergoing coronary artery bypass grafting having an EF ≤35%, and an abnormal signal-averaged ECG. Nine hundred patients were randomized to receive either an ICD or no ICD at the time of clinically indicated elective coronary artery bypass surgery. Over an average follow-up of 32 months, the actuarial total mortality rates in the control and ICD therapy groups were 24% and 27%, respectively ($p = 0.64$). Although patients randomized to ICD therapy experienced a 45% lower rate of deaths attributed to arrhythmia than the control group ($p = 0.057$), the rate of nonarrhythmic cardiac deaths did not differ between the two treatment groups.[34]

The DINAMIT trial was the first to specifically target patients with recent MI.[32] In this study, 674 patients with an infarction 6–40 days earlier, having an EF ≤35%, and a marker of autonomic dysfunction (either abnormal heart rate variability or an elevated average heart rate over 24 hours on Holter monitor) were randomized equally to a control group without specific anti-arrhythmic therapy versus the active treatment group that received an ICD. After an average follow-up of 30 months, the patients randomized to ICD therapy had fewer deaths attributable to arrhythmia, but significantly greater non-arrhythmic deaths. There was no significant difference in total mortality between the two treatment groups. It is important to recognize the fact that a majority of patients in each treatment group received (appropriate) therapy with β-blocking agents and ACE-inhibitors.

The rationale behind the recommendation that ICDs not be implanted within 40 days after AMI has several bases. First, EF usually increases after AMI, in part dependent on whether and when reperfusion occurs. Thus, measurement of EF within 2 weeks of AMI is not likely to represent the true, stable value of EF. A minority of patients in the MUSTT and MADIT trials were enrolled within the first month after MI. Thus, these studies do not address the utility of ICDs applied within this time frame. Second, a substudy analysis of patients enrolled into the MADIT II study showed that patients enrolled into that trial within 17 months of AMI experienced no improvement in survival with ICD treatment.[35] Finally, the DINAMIT trial showed no improvement in survival when ICDs were implanted within 40 days after AMI.

It has been recognized for some time that patients with congestive heart failure due to LV systolic dysfunction, regardless of etiology (both coronary disease as well as nonischemic dilated cardiomyopathy) are at high risk for sudden death. Although at least 50% of patients enrolled in all the aforementioned trials had a history of symptomatic heart failure, the issue of whether patients with a primary diagnosis of congestive heart failure given contemporary medical therapy might benefit from ICD therapy was unclear. In addition, the role of ICDs for primary prevention of sudden death in patients with heart failure due to nonischemic dilated cardiomyopathy was unknown until recently. Two recent small-randomized trials have evaluated the ICD versus conventional therapy in patients with heart failure due to nonischemic dilated cardiomyopathy, while a third large study enrolled patients with congestive heart failure congestive heart failure (CHF) with either ischemic or nonischemic mediated LV dysfunction.

The Cardiomyopathy Trial (CAT) enrolled 104 patients with idiopathic dilated cardiomyopathy diagnosed within 9 months, EF ≤30%, and NYHA Class II or III.[36] The mean EF was 24%. After a mean follow-up of 5.5 years, no difference in survival emerged between the two treatment groups. The mortality rates were very low in each group: total mortality at 2-year follow-up was 8% in the ICD treated patients versus 7% in the control group. These event rates are markedly lower than those observed in the primary prevention studies of patients with coronary artery disease discussed earlier. A second trial, Defibrillators in Nonischemic Cardiomyopathy Treatment Evaluation ("DEFINITE"), randomized 458 patients with nonischemic dilated cardiomyopathy to standard medical therapy alone, or combined with an ICD.[37] The average EF of enrolled patients was 21%, and the majority of patients were on β-blockers and ACE-inhibitors. After a mean follow-up of 29 months, no significant difference in survival was noted between the two treatment groups. Total mortality at 2 years was 14.1% in the patients randomized to standard therapy versus 7.9% in the ICD group (hazard ratio 0.65, $p = 0.08$). The risk of deaths attributed to arrhythmia was significantly lower in the ICD-treated patients (hazard ratio 0.20, $p = 0.0006$).

Finally, the role of the ICD in patients with congestive heart failure has been addressed by the Sudden Cardiac Death in Heart Failure Trial (SCD-HeFT).[28] This trial enrolled 2521 patients with NYHA Class II or III symptoms, an EF ≤35% due to either coronary disease ($N = 1310$ patients) or nonischemic dilated cardiomyopathy ($N = 1211$ patients). The design of this study incorporated three treatment arms: placebo, amiodarone, or ICD. After a mean follow-up of 45.5 months, there was no significant difference in survival between the placebo and amiodarone treated group. The 2-year mortality in the placebo group was 14.5%. In contrast, the 2-year mortality of patients randomized to the ICD was 11.6% (hazard ratio 0.77, $p = 0.007$ in comparison to placebo). In this study, improved survival was observed in ICD treated patients, regardless of the etiology of CHF.

A number of conditions exist for which it is recognized that the ICD is not indicated at present. These include ventricular tachyarrhythmias for which primary cures exist, such as those associated with rapid atrial tachycardias in patients with Wolff–Parkinson–White Syndrome, VT due to transient or reversible disorders, and idiopathic VT curable by radiofrequency catheter ablation (noted previously). A second group of conditions for which ICDs are not indicated are those in which the ICD would not improve the patients' survival or overall quality of life. These include incessant VT or VF, significant psychiatric illnesses that could be aggravated by ICD discharges or that preclude adequate ICD follow-up care, terminal illnesses, and Class IV refractory congestive heart failure patients, who are not candidates for cardiac transplantation.

In conclusion, multiple well-designed clinical trials have now clearly demonstrated the ability of the ICD to reduce the risk of arrhythmic death and overall mortality in selected patient populations. It is likely that there will be significant growth in the utilization of ICDs for primary prevention of sudden death in the future. In fact, future growth for this indication may well outpace growth in the number of devices implanted for secondary prevention. The challenge for physicians at this time is better risk stratification to define the patients who are likely to derive the most benefit from this therapy.

References

1 Mirowski M, Reid P, Mower M. Termination of malignant ventricular arrhythmias with an implanted automatic defibrillator in human beings. *N Engl J Med* 1980; 303: 322–4.

2 Ruskin JN, Camm AJ, Zipes DP *et al.* Implantable cardioverter defibrillator utilization based on discharge diagnoses from Medicare and managed care patients. *J Cardiovasc Electrophysiol* 2002; 13: 38–43.

3 Baum R, Alvarez H, Cobb LA. Survival after resuscitation from out-of-hospital ventricular fibrillation. *Circulation* 1974; 50: 1231–5.

4 The Antiarrhythmics versus Implantable Defibrillators (AVID) Investigators. A comparison of antiarrhythmic-drug therapy with implantable defibrillators in patients resuscitated from near-fatal ventricular arrhythmias. *N Engl J Med* 1997; 337: 1576–83.

5 Domanski M, Saksena S, Epstein A *et al.* Relative effectiveness of the implantable cardioverter-defibrillator and antiarrhythmic drugs in patients with varying degrees of left ventricular dysfunction who have survived malignant ventricular arrhythmias. *J Am Coll Cardiol* 1999; 34: 1090–5.

6 Raitt MH, Dolack GL, Kudenchuk PJ *et al.* Ventricular arrhythmias detected after transvenous defibrillator implantation in patients with a clinical history of only ventricular fibrillation. Implications for use of implantable defibrillator. *Circulation* 1995; 91: 1996–2001.

7 Bansch D, Castrucci M, Bocker D *et al.* Ventricular tachycardias above the initially programmed tachycardia detection interval in patients with implantable cardioverter-defibrillators: incidence, prediction and significance. *J Am Coll Cardiol* 2000; 36: 557–65.

8 Kuck K-H, Cappato R, Siebels J *et al.* Randomized comparison of antiarrhythmic drug therapy with implantable defibrillators in patients resuscitated from cardiac arrest. The Cardiac Arrest Study Hamburg (CASH). *Circulation* 2000; 102: 748–54.

9 Connolly S, Gent M, Roberts R *et al.* Canadian Implantable Defibrillator Study (CIDS) – A randomized trial of the implantable cardioverter defibrillator against amiodarone. *Circulation* 2000; 101: 1297–1302.

10 Connolly SJ, Hallstrom AP, Cappato R *et al.* Meta-analysis of the implantable cardioverter defibrillator secondary prevention trials. *Eur Heart J* 2000; 21: 2071–8.

11 Wyse DG, Friedman PL, Brodsky MA *et al.* Life-threatening ventricular arrhythmias due to transient or correctable causes: High risk for death in follow-up. *J Am Coll Cardiol* 2001; 38: 1718–24.

12 Volpi A, Cavalli A, Santoro L *et al.* Incidence and prognosis of early primary ventricular fibrillation in acute myocardial infarction — results of the Gruppo Italiano per lo Studio della Sopravivenza nell'Infarto Miocardico (GISSI-2) database. *Am J Cardiol* 1998; 82: 265–71.

13 Goldberg R, Gore J, Haffajee C *et al.* Outcome after cardiac arrest during acute myocardial infarction. *Am J Cardiol* 1987; 59: 251–5.

14 Behar S, Goldbourt U, Reicher-Reiss H *et al.* Prognosis of acute myocardial infarction complicated by primary ventricular fibrillation. *Am J Cardiol* 1990; 66: 1208–11.

15 Brugada J, Aguinaga L, Mont L *et al.* Coronary artery revascularization in patients with sustained ventricular arrhythmias in the chronic phase of a myocardial infarction: effects on the electrophysiologic substrate and outcome [comment]. *J Am Coll Cardiol* 2001; 37: 529–33.

16 Natale A, Sra J, Axtell K *et al.* Ventricular fibrillation and polymorphic ventricular tachycardia with critical coronary artery stenosis: Does bypass surgery suffice? *J Cardiovasc Electrophysiol* 1994; 5: 988–94.

17 Brugada P, Talajic M, Smeets J *et al.* The value of the clinical history to assess prognosis of patients with ventricular tachycardia or ventricular fibrillation after myocardial infarction. *Eur Heart J* 1989; 10: 747–52.

18 Sarter BH, Finkle JK, Gerszten RE *et al.* What is the risk of sudden cardiac death in patients presenting with hemodynamically stable sustained ventricular tachycardia after myocardial infarction? *J Am Coll Cardiol* 1996; 28: 122–9.

19 Raitt MH, Renfroe EG, Epstein AE *et al.* "Stable" ventricular tachycardia is not a benign rhythm: insights from the antiarrhythmics versus implantable defibrillators (AVID) registry. *Circulation* 2001; 103: 244–52.

20 Blanck Z, Deshpande S, Jazayeri M *et al.* Catheter ablation of the left bundle branch for the treatment of sustained bundle branch reentrant ventricular tachycardia. *J Cardiovasc Electrophysiol* 1995; 6: 40–3.

21 Middlekauff HR, Stevenson WG, Stevenson LW *et al.* Syncope in advanced heart failure: high risk of sudden death regardless of origin of syncope. *J Am Coll Cardiol* 1993; 21: 110–6.

22 Fonarow G, Feliciano Z, Boyle N *et al.* Improved survival in patients with nonischemic advanced heart failure and syncope treated with an implantable cardioverter-defibrillator. *Am J Cardiol* 2000; 85: 981–5.

23 Knight B, Goyal R, Pelosi F *et al.* Outcome of patients with nonischemic dilated cardiomyopathy and unexplained syncope treated with an implantable defibrillator. *J Am Coll Cardiol* 1999; 33: 1964–70.

24 Zheng Z-J, Croft JB, Giles WH *et al.* Sudden cardiac death in the United States, 1989 to 1998. *Circulation* 2001; 104: 2158–63.

25 Myerburg RJ, Fenster J, Velez M *et al.* Impact of community-wide police car deployment of automated external defibrillators on survival from out-of-hospital cardiac arrest. *Circulation* 2002; 106: 1058–64.

26 Buxton AE, Fisher JD, Josephson ME *et al.* Prevention of sudden death in patients with coronary artery disease: the Multicenter Unsustained Tachycardia Trial (MUSTT). *Prog Cardiovasc Dis* 1993; 36: 215–26.

27 Moss AJ, Zareba W, Hall WJ *et al.* Prophylactic implantation of a defibrillator in patients with myocardial infarction and reduced ejection fraction. *N Engl J Med* 2002; 346: 877–83.

28 Bardy GH, Lee KL, Mark DB *et al.* Amiodarone or an implantable cardioverter-defibrillator for congestive heart failure. *N Engl J Med* 2005; 352: 225–37.

29 Bigger J, The Coronary Artery Bypass Graft (CABG) Patch Trial Investigators. Prophylactic use of implanted cardiac defibrillators in patients at high risk for ventricular arrhythmias after coronary-artery bypass graft surgery. *N Engl J Med* 1997; 337: 1569–75.

30 Moss AJ, Hall WJ, Cannom DS *et al.* Improved survival with an implanted defibrillator in patients with coronary disease at high risk for ventricular arrhythmia. Multicenter Automatic Defibrillator Implantation Trial Investigators. *N Engl J Med* 1996; 335: 1933–40.

31 Buxton AE, Lee KL, Fisher JD *et al.* A randomized study of the prevention of sudden death in patients with coronary artery disease. *N Engl J Med* 1999; 341: 1882–90.

32 Hohnloser SH, Kuck KH, Dorian P *et al.* Prophylactic use of an implantable cardioverter-defibrillator after acute myocardial infarction. *N Engl J Med* 2004; 351: 2481–8.

33 Lee KL, Hafley G, Fisher JD *et al.* Effect of implantable defibrillators on arrhythmic events and mortality in the multicenter unsustained tachycardia trial. *Circulation* 2002; 106: 233–8.

34 Bigger JT, Whang W, Rottman JN *et al.* Mechanisms of death in the CABG Patch trial. *Circulation* 1999; 99: 1416–21.

35 Wilbur D, Zareba W, Hall W *et al.* Time dependence of mortality risk and defibrillator benefit after myocardial infarction. *Circulation* 2004; 109: 1082–4.

36 Bansch D, Antz M, Boczor S *et al.* Primary prevention of sudden cardiac death in idiopathic dilated cardiomyopathy: The Cardiomyopathy Trial (CAT). *Circulation* 2002; 105: 1453–8.

37 Kadish A, Dyer A, Daubert J *et al.* Prophylactic defibrillator implantation in patients with nonschemic dilated cardiomyopathy. *N Engl J Med* 2004; 350: 2151–8.

CHAPTER 6

ICD follow-up: complications, troubleshooting, and emergencies related to ICDs

Kristin E. Ellison

The implantable cardioverter-defibrillator (ICD) has been established as an effective treatment for prevention of sudden cardiac death. ICD indications continue to expand and the number of ICD implants continues to grow exponentially. This chapter reviews current practice guidelines for ICD follow-up and complications related to device implants; it also provides an update on stored diagnostic data that provide crucial information about device function, arrhythmia documentation, and enable troubleshooting of problems related to ICD function. Emergencies related to ICDs are also reviewed, as well as the management of the ICD patient during the perioperative period. Electromagnetic interference (EMI) and hospital sources of interference are discussed, as well as the psychological aspects of defibrillator implantation to the patient.

Perioperative management

The most common intraoperative and immediate postoperative complications of the ICD implant include pneumothorax, hemothorax, lead penetration or perforation with possible resultant cardiac tamponade, device pocket hematoma, brachial plexus injury, arterial puncture, venous thrombosis, and complications related to surgical anesthesia.

The immediate postimplantation follow-up is focused on the surgical aspects of device implantation. Standard practice is to keep the wound dry for at least a week to avoid contamination of the incision by skin bacteria. The patient should be evaluated 1 to 2 weeks after implantation for inspection of the wound to assess for evidence of a seroma, hematoma, or infection.

We advise patients not to perform any activity more strenuous than walking for at least 1 month after implant. Patients should avoid heavy lifting using the arm on the side of the defibrillator. In addition, we advise limiting the range of motion of this arm to avoid excessive force on the lead. In this regard, patients should refrain from driving until the leads are secure. This recommendation is for those patients who have the device implanted for primary prevention (i.e., they have not had a prior arrhythmic event). For patients with devices implanted after a cardiac arrest or syncopal ventricular tachycardia (VT) (secondary prevention), the driving restrictions vary from state to state in the United States, but the general recommendation is to refrain from driving for at least 6 months. Initial visits to the physician should also be dedicated to patient education regarding the defibrillator, as well as to the reassurance of the patient.

In the Multicenter Automatic Defibrillator Implantation trial II (MADIT II), 742 patients received implantable defibrillators.[1] Serious complications related to defibrillator therapy were infrequent. No deaths occurred during implantation, 1.8% of patients had lead-related complications, and there were five nonfatal infections (0.7%) that required surgical intervention. In the Antiarrhythmic versus Implantable Defibrillator (AVID) trial, 93% of the device implants were nonthoracotomy implants. The overall rate of infection was 10 out of 507 implants or 1.9%.[2] In the Multicenter unsustained Tachycardia Trial (MUSST) there was one fatal infection out of 161 implants.[3]

Routine follow-up

Once the wound has healed, patients should be seen at regular intervals to monitor the implantation site, assess the device function, and review detections of arrhythmia and delivered therapies.[4] The follow-up interval ranges between 1 and 6 months, depending on the patient's condition. Patients may need to be seen more frequently to evaluate the efficacy of drug therapy, and assess the burden of both atrial and ventricular arrhythmias. The goals of the defibrillator patient's follow-up are outlined in Box 6.1.[5] The cardiac status and general health of the patient must also be reviewed, as many patients have concomitant cardiac problems such as congestive heart failure or coronary artery disease.

As with pacemaker therapy, a major objective of follow-up is to maximize device longevity. Device longevity varies considerably between manufacturers, but is related to the extent of bradycardia pacing, frequency and energy of delivered shocks, and extent of data collection and storage.[6] When lead function has stabilized, approximately 3 months after implant, pacing

---

Box 6.1   Goals of the defibrillator patient's follow-up

- Recording the nature and frequency of arrhythmias
- Identification and recording of device activity
- Assessment of pacing and sensing functions
- Assessment of battery status
- Enhancement of pulse generator longevity
- Optimization of therapeutic parameters based on the device history
- Optimization of ancillary parameters, such as diagnostic enhancements
- Assessment of general cardiac status

outputs should be decreased to provide a two- to three-fold safety margin over threshold to preserve battery life. The extent of safety margin depends on whether a patient is pacer dependent or not. Patients who do not require pacing may have their devices programmed with a lower safety margin (1.5–2 times threshold).

In patients with preserved intrinsic atrioventricular (AV) conduction, the AV delay interval (the time between atrial events and ventricular pacing) should be prolonged to avoid right ventricular (RV) pacing. Right ventricular apical pacing results in differential timing of contraction between the right and left ventricle, analogous to left bundle branch block physiology that results in less efficient ventricular contraction.[7] This may worsen heart failure in patients with depressed left ventricular (LV) function, as shown in the Dual chamber VVI Implantable Defibrillator (DAVID) trial and even in patients with preserved LV function, as documented in the Mode Selection Trial (MOST) trial.[8,9] Therefore, prolonging the AV interval to allow an intrinsic AV conduction with a narrow QRS is beneficial for cardiac function, as well as device longevity.

An essential aspect of defibrillator patient follow-up is the identification and recording of tachyarrhythmias and the device treatment of these arrhythmias. Newer ICDs contain detailed data storage capabilities. This includes event marker channels and intracardiac electrograms (Figure 6.1). These features enable the physician to determine if ICD therapy was appropriate (i.e. for VT/VF) or inappropriate (e.g. sinus tachycardia, SVT, or oversensing cardiac

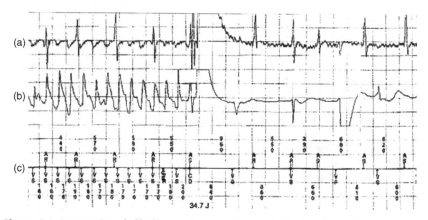

Figure 6.1 Appropriate defibrillation therapy. Tracing (a) is the atrial electrogram. Tracing (b) is the ventricular electrogram, and tracing (c) is the marker channel. The figure demonstrates ventricular fibrillation; note greater number of ventricular events than atrial events. The atrial cycle length ranges between 440 and 580 ms (number between atrial events on marker channel). Events labeled AR fall in the atrial refractory period. Ventricular events occur with a cycle length of 160 to 180 ms. CD denotes charge delivered, resulting in sinus rhythm, with occasional ventricular and atrial ectopy. Note evidence of far-field R-wave sensing on the atrial channel, but this does not register an atrial event on the marker channel. A 34.7 J shock terminates ventricular fibrillation.

and noncardiac events, such as lead noise). Newer defibrillators provide tabulated chronological diagnostic data recordings and lead function. Devices can take periodic measurements of lead impedance, pacing thresholds, battery voltage, charge times, capacitor reformation times, high voltage lead impedance, and frequency and timing of VTs, allowing for early detection of lead insulation breaks, fractures, dislodgment, and other problems. The analysis of stored electrograms may also alert the physician to unrecognized atrial arrhythmias and the need for anticoagulation. Diagnostic data may provide the rationale for institution or change of an antiarrhythmic drug therapy, or reprogramming such as the addition of antitachycardia pacing. Devices may also be programmed to provide patient alerts, which emit an audible tone when certain parameter values are obtained; the most important of these would be an elective replacement indicator determined by the battery status. Typically, devices are designed to operate for an additional 3 months even after tripping of the elective replacement indicator. However, battery life may be erratic at its end-of-life. Therefore, it is important to replace the pulse generator at the first opportunity after the elective replacement indicator is reached.

Lead complications

Initial lead concerns relate to lead dislodgment and its connection to the ICD (often resulting from failure to adequately tighten the set screw that fastens the lead to the generator). Routine device follow-up may reveal evidence of "micro" or overt lead dislodgment, exit block, insulation breaches, conductor coil fractures, and lead infection. These and other lead complications are reviewed in Chapter 9. A baseline chest X-ray (posteroanterior and lateral) is routinely obtained after device implantation for comparison with subsequent chest X-rays. Some centers obtain chest X-rays on an annual basis, other centers only when a problem is suspected.

Defibrillation threshold testing

The amount of energy required to reproducibly terminate ventricular fibrillation is termed the defibrillation threshold (DFT). DFT testing is performed at device implant, unless there are compelling reasons not to, such as embolic risks (in some patients with atrial fibrillation), recent coronary intervention, and concern regarding transient cerebral hypoperfusion. Our practice is to repeat DFT testing at 3 months when lead function has stabilized. The need for DFT testing at regular intervals after implantation is somewhat controversial. Arrhythmia detection and effective treatment cannot be assessed during a routine device interrogation. Annual DFT testing may suggest the need for device reprogramming to provide effective first shock therapy and occasionally will uncover device malfunction, which requires surgical intervention. This is particularly true with abdominal devices after second generator replacements (Personal communication, M.O. Sweeney, MD).

Table 6.1 Effects of antiarrhythmic drugs on DFT

Drug class	Drug	Effect on DFT
IA	Quinidine	↔
	Disopyramide	↔
	Procainamide	↔
IB	Lidocaine	↑
	Phenytoin	↑
	Mexiletine	↑, ↔
IC	Flecainide	↑
	Propafenone	↓
II	Propranolol	↑
	Timolol	↔
III	Amiodarone	↑
	Sotalol	↓
	Bretylium	↔

↔= neutral; ↑= increase; ↓= decrease.

Many patients with implantable defibrillators require adjunctive antiarrhythmic drug therapy. Drug therapy may be initiated in general to suppress frequent episodes of ventricular tachycardia or supraventricular tachyarrhythmias, especially if these result in an ICD shock. Antiarrhythmic drugs may help to slow the rate of VT. This in turn often enables overdrive pacing (ATP) to terminate VT, avoiding shock therapy. Some antiarrhythmic agents may affect both pacing and DFTS. Table 6.1 outlines the effect of various antiarrhythmic drugs on DFTs.[10] Newer ICDs have noninvasive means of assessing high-voltage lead integrity. It is the policy at our institution to test devices after initiation of amiodarone, as it commonly increases the energy requirements for defibrillation. We also routinely retest patients who have had a failed first shock therapy and annually test patients whose defibrillation threshold does not provide a 10 J safety margin, that is, DFT >20 J in a device whose maximum device output is 30 J.

Management of patients who have received device therapies

Patients who report a single shock without sequelae, can be evaluated with routine office visits, preferably seen within 48 hours. However, patients receiving multiple shocks within a short period should contact their physicians immediately, and if patients have complaints of chest pain, dizziness, or difficulty in breathing, they should call for emergency evaluation (i.e. 911 in the United States). In older ICDs, the appropriateness of therapy was determined largely on the basis of symptoms prior to the shock. We now appreciate that the presence or absence of symptoms prior to delivery of therapy is not very helpful in determining the etiology (or appropriateness) of a shock. ICDs now respond so rapidly to ventricular tachyarrhythmias that symptoms prior to shock are not always present, and it is not unusual in patients with ventricular fibrillation to have a shock as their only symptom of the event. Many patients with VT deny awareness of palpitations before ICD therapy. Prolonged symptoms such as palpitations, dizziness, chest pain, or shortness of breath warrant immediate evaluation, and may represent issues such as device undersensing or inappropriate detection rates for VT and ventricular fibrillation. In addition, this may represent battery depletion with prolonged charge times of the defibrillator.

Multiple shocks

Multiple ICD shocks in a short period of time constitute a medical emergency. They may result from recurrent ventricular arrhythmias (ventricular electrical "storm"), supraventricular arrhythmias, or ICD system malfunctions. Multiple shocks produce profound psychological morbidity. Many patients become anxious and agitated.[11] When multiple shocks result from ICD system failure, rapid identification of the problem may be life saving. Multiple shocks also result in substantial battery depletion. The causes of repeated ICD shocks are multifactorial, and interpretation of stored electrograms can be crucial to identification of the etiology. ICD firings may effectively terminate a ventricular arrhythmia followed by prompt reinitiation. Devices may also fail to defibrillate. This may result from inadequate shock energies, that is, therapies being programmed below the DFT. Addition of antiarrhythmic agents may increase DFT energy. Leads may migrate or structurally break down. Up to 10% of patients receive spurious ICD shocks in response to supraventricular arrhythmias, most often atrial fibrillation or sinus tachycardia.[12] This may be avoided by programming SVT discriminators as outlined in Chapter 7.

The patient's clinical status must be assessed whenever a shock has been delivered. This is especially critical when a patient receives multiple shocks. Inquiry should be made for recent chest pain, suggestive of myocardial ischemia. Electrolyte abnormalities may also result in myocardial irritability. These may reflect drug-induced proarrhythmia, such as prolonged QT and *torsade de pointes*. Recurrent VT may also be precipitated by congestive heart failure. Patients with incessant or frequent tachycardias, in spite of antiarrhythmic drug treatment should be considered for ablation of the VT. Multiple ICD shocks have been associated with a small release of myocardial enzymes in the absence of other evidence of myocardial infarction.[13]

False arrhythmia detection

Oversensing by a device relates to inappropriate sensing of electrical signals, and may result in false event detection. Oversensing may result in inhibition of

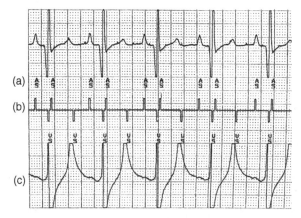

Figure 6.2 Real-time recording during sinus rhythm. Panel (a) is surface telemetry, panel (b) is the marker channel and panel (c) is the ventricular electrogram. AS denotes atrial sensed events, VS denotes ventricular sensed events. The marker channel demonstrates double counting on both atrial and ventricular channels. The atrial channel is oversensing far-field R-waves and the ventricular channel is oversensing the T-wave.

pacing, inappropriate mode switching, or inappropriate ICD tachyarrhythmia detections with possible therapy delivery. The causes of oversensing may be determined by analysis of real time and stored electrograms with event markers. Oversensing of intrinsic events can be identified through device interrogation. There may be oversensing of depolarization events (such as P and R waves) or repolarization events (T-wave oversensing). Oversensing of depolarization events can result from sensing events occurring in another cardiac chamber, such as sensing ventricular events on the atrial channel or vice versa (far-field oversensing). Far-field oversensing of atrial signals on the ventricular channel of an ICD may trigger false tachyarrhythmias detection. Figure 6.2 demonstrates T-wave oversensing on the ventricular lead, as well as far-field R-wave sensing on the atrial lead.

T-wave oversensing is a common problem seen in ICDs. This may be related to the absolute size of the T-wave, or the size of the depolarization R-wave relative to the T-wave. This is a dynamic relationship that can be altered by metabolic conditions (electrolytes, ischemia, as well as after an ICD shock delivery). In one large series, T-wave oversensing was much more frequently seen on leads with larger sensing "antenna" (integrated bipolar leads) versus leads with a smaller "antenna" (true bipolar leads).[14] Reprogramming may be necessary to adjust signal detection sensitivity to avoid T-wave sensing. However, it is as crucial to ensure that there is adequate device detection of ventricular arrhythmias if the device sensitivity is decreased to avoid T-wave sensing. T-wave oversensing in the ventricle may also be corrected by reprogramming (prolonging) the ventricular refractory period.

Office evaluation of patients after frequent shocks

It is important to know the device manufacturer and implant date, lead locations, antiarrhythmic drug history, as well as presence or absence of symptoms of heart failure or angina, preceding device therapies. Certain leads or devices may be subject to alert status. Certain lead models are known to have premature insulation breakdown.[15] It can be useful to have the patient reenact whatever body position was associated with shock occurrence while monitoring the implanted device through the programmer. This is best done when the device therapy has been deactivated, to avoid an inappropriate therapy if there is a suspicion of false detection. Physical manipulation of the ICD generator pocket may elicit noise related to a loose set screw. Vagal maneuvers, as well as deep inspiration, may elicit diaphragmatic oversensing (i.e. sensing myopotentials generated by diaphragmatic contraction). This is particularly prominent in patients who have leads with more widely spaced electrodes (resulting in a larger sensing "antenna") coupled with the devices that have more aggressive signal gain functions.[16]

Problems related to biventricular devices

There are unique sensing issues related to biventricular devices, especially older Y adapted and Guidant systems that had both RV and LV sensing that can lead to double counting of ventricular events. These problems are now rarely seen with newer models with separate ports for right and left leads, sensing only from the RV lead and synchronous biventricular pacing.

Device–Device interaction

Previously, ICDs and pacemakers were implanted separately in patients who required atrial pacing for bradycardia and a defibrillator. This is no longer the case, as modern ICDs incorporate sophisticated pacing functions. When patients do have separate pacemakers and defibrillators, careful testing is required to ensure adequate arrhythmia detection and post-shock pacer function.[17] Box 6.2 summarizes potential pacemaker and ICD interactions.[18]

Device malfunction

ICD malfunction is uncommon. Inappropriate therapy or absence of expected therapy most often relates to inappropriate device programming. Other factors, such as lead related complications, drug/device interactions, or device–device (pacemaker/ICD) interactions in patients with separate implanted devices lacking diagnostic specificity (particularly with single chamber ICDs) are also common. True device component malfunction is very rare, but must be considered when no other explanation can be found.

> **Box 6.2 Potential pacemaker and implantable cardioverter-defibrillator (ICD) interactions**
>
> *Pacemaker – ICD interactions*
>   VF nondetection because of pacemaker stimuli
>   Especially a problem with unipolar pacemakers
>   Double, triple, and multiple counting, resulting in false positive shocks
> *ICD – pacemaker interactions*
>   Pacemaker reprogramming because of ICD discharge
>   Sensing and capture failure after defibrillation
> *ICD – antitachycardia pacemaker interactions*
>   Antitachycardia pacing triggering ICD discharges

Device identification/magnet function

Rapid identification of an ICD model may be important when it is necessary to deactivate or reprogram a patient's device. Patients should be instructed to carry identification cards that identify the manufacturer generator model and lead system. This is particularly important, as there is not a universal programmer for all ICDs, and each device will only respond to a manufacturer-specific program. If the manufacturer is unknown, an overpenetrated chest X-ray over the device pocket may show marks on the pulse generator that will identify the vendor. When a specific programmer is not available, a magnet may be placed on top of all ICD models to temporarily disable arrhythmia detection. The magnetic field closes a reed switch in the generator circuit. In general, as long as the magnet remains in close proximity to the pulse generator, tachyarrhythmia recognition and treatment is disabled. There will be no effect on pacing function.

Electromagnetic interference

Pacemakers and ICDs are both subject to interference from nonbiologic electromagnetic sources.[19] Modern ICDs are shielded from most sources of interference by the stainless steel or titanium case. ICDs also have bipolar or integrated bipolar leads that decrease the range of the sensing antenna to help shield against EMI. EMI enters the ICD by conduction, if the patient is in direct contact, or by radiation, if the patient is in the electromagnetic field with the lead acting as an antenna. The electromagnetic spectrum that impacts implantable devices includes frequencies between 0 and 109 Hz, such as alternating current electricity supplies (50–60 Hz), as well as electrocautery (radiofrequencies at approximately 500 kHz). These signals may be interpreted as cardiac signals and inappropriately inhibit or trigger device responses, such as inappropriate inhibition of paced outputs, inappropriate triggering of paced outputs, asynchronous pacing, reprogramming (usually to a back-up mode),

---

Box 6.3   Sources of EMI in the hospital environment

- Electrocautery
- Cardioversion, defibrillation
- MRI
- Lithotripsy
- Radiofrequency ablation
- Electroshock therapy
- Electroconvulsive therapy
- Diathermy

---

or damage to device circuitry, triggering an ICD discharge. High intensity therapeutic X-rays, as well as therapeutic ultrasound, may also damage device circuitry directly. When defibrillators are in the field of a therapeutic radiation, we generally utilize lead extenders to enable relocation of the device out of the targeted area.

The principal sources of EMI that affect devices are found in the hospital environment, and are listed in Box 6.3.[20] Electrocautery during surgical procedures is a common source. ICDs are likely to interpret the electrocautery as ventricular fibrillation, triggering shock therapy. Device circuitry can also be damaged. Patients undergoing procedures requiring cautery should have their devices interrogated prior to the procedure. Programmed settings should be recorded, and the underlying rhythm should be determined. Tachycardia detection should be disabled just before surgery and restored immediately after surgery. Under these circumstances, it is critical that the patient have back-up external defibrillation available. An alternate approach is to place a magnet over the device during surgery. This approach has the advantage of allowing the anesthesiologist or surgeon to remove the magnet, if the patient develops tachyarrhythmias intraoperatively. The magnet feature does not affect the pacemaker function of the defibrillator, and electrocautery may still result in inhibition of pacer output intraoperatively. In this case, short bursts of minimally effective current with electrocautery are recommended. The closer the cautery probe is to the pulse generator, the greater the risk of adverse interaction. This is especially important to remember during head, neck, shoulder, and thoracic procedures. Postoperatively, the device should be reinterrogated and reprogrammed appropriately. Pacing thresholds should be reassessed and compared with preoperative values. Radiofrequency catheter ablation has the same effects as coagulation electrocautery, and similar precautions should be utilized.

External thoracic defibrillation or cardioversion produces the largest amount of electrical energy delivered in the vicinity of a device. It has the potential to damage both pulse generator and cardiac tissue in contact with the lead. Therefore, during cardioversion or defibrillation, the paddles should be placed as far from the pulse generator as possible. The device should be interrogated after the procedure.

Implanted defibrillators constitute a strong contraindication to Magnetic Resonance Imaging (MRI), as this has been known to cause serious pacemaker and defibrillator malfunction.[20] Exposure to a magnetic field occurs on entry into the MRI suite. This may result in suspension of tachyarrhythmia detection. The static magnetic field can also impart rotational and translational forces to the generator. Newer ICD models may become more MRI compatible (tolerant). However, at this time, ICDs remain a contraindication to the use of MRI imaging.

Other hospital sources of interference include extracorporeal shock wave lithotripsy for the treatment of nephrolithiasis and cholelithiasis. Transcutaneous electrical nerve stimulation may affect device function, and it is reasonable to test the unit under a monitored setting prior to having the patient utilize such devices at home.

Community-based EMI influences include cellular telephone, electronic article surveillance, power stations, arc welding equipment, CB and ham radio equipment, and automobile ignition systems. Microwave ovens are no longer considered significant sources of interference. Antitheft devices in many department stores involve an electronic field that senses an electronic tag as the customer exits through the gate. It is generally recommended that patients pass quickly through the gates to avoid any interference related to the magnetic field. The incidence of interference from cellular phones is variable between the different manufacturers. Cellular phones using digital technology are reported to have greater possibility of device interference.[21] It is generally recommended that patients utilize the cell phone on the side opposite from their pulse generator. Interference increases with increasing proximity to the device generator.

Device infection

An ICD system infection represents a potentially lethal complication. Infections are more common after generator replacement. Device infection and lead extraction are discussed in Chapter 9.

Ethical and psychological aspects of defibrillators

The presence of an ICD in the terminally ill patient raises medical and ethical issues. Deactivation of the ICD is appropriate when the device is believed to prolong the patient's suffering. This must be discussed with the patient, family, and primary physician. Any decision to deactivate an ICD must be documented appropriately, with explicit consent being obtained.

The psychological aspects of ICD therapy have been studied.[22] ICD shock therapy, although therapeutic, may be perceived as highly adverse by patients. Anxiety and vigilant monitoring of physical symptoms are common among ICD patients. Estimates of anxiety related to ICD shock among patients vary, with up to 50% of patients experiencing anxiety. Panic disorders and agoraphobia may occur after ICD implantation. In one study, 16% of patients experienced agoraphobia or panic disorder after ICD implantation, and 14% showed functional avoidance that did not meet criteria for a panic disorder. Functional avoidance that is not medically recommended is common among patients with ICDs. This may have adverse effects on quality of life, and perhaps the physical health of some patients.[22] A brief educational intervention or regular participation in ICD support groups can help dispel misinformation among patients, discourage inappropriate avoidance, and provide a greater sense of well being.[23]

ICDs can prolong survival in selected patients, yet devices are not without risk. These risks must be taken into account and discussed with patients prior to implantation. They become especially important when implanting ICDs prophylactically for primary prevention.

References

1 Moss AJ, Zareba W, Hall WJ. Prophylactic implantation of a defibrillator in patients with myocardial infarction and reduced ejection fraction. *N Engl J Med* 2002; 346: 877–83.

2 Zipes D, Wyse DG, Friedman PL *et al.* A comparison of antiarrhythmic drug therapy with implantable defibrillators in patients resuscitated from near-fatal ventricular arrhythmias. *N Engl J Med* 1997; 337: 1576–83.

3 Buxton AE, Lee KL, Fisher JD *et al.* A randomized study of the prevention of sudden death in patients with coronary artery disease. *N Engl J Med* 1999; 341: 1882–90.

4 DiMarco JP. Medical progress: implantable cardioverter-defibrillators. *N Engl J Med* 2003; 349: 1836–47.

5 Crossley GH. Follow-up of the patient with a defibrillator, in Ellenbogen KA, Kay GN, and Wilkoff BL (eds). *Cardiac Pacing and Defibrillation*. Philadelphia: W.B. Saunders, 2000, pp. 931–938.

6 Karasik P, Steele P, Ellenbogen KA *et al.* Longevity variation for implantable defibrillators in the VA Database. *Circulation* 1996; 94: I-563.

7 Grines CL, Bashore TM, Boudoulas H *et al.* Functional abnormalities in isolated left bundle branch block: the effect of interventricular asynchrony. *Circulation* 1989; 79: 845–53.

8 Wilkoff BL, Cook JR, Epstein AE *et al.* Dual-chamber pacing or ventricular backup pacing in patients with an implantable defibrillator: the Dual Chamber and VVI Implantable Defibrillator (DAVID) Trial. *JAMA* 2002; 288: 3115–23.

9 Sweeney MO, Hellkamp AS, Ellenbogen KA *et al.* Adverse effect of ventricular pacing on heart failure and atrial fibrillation among patients with normal baseline QRS duration in a clinical trial of pacemaker therapy for sinus node dysfunction. *Circulation* 2003; 107: 2932–7.

10 Gollob MH, Seger JJ. Current status of the implantable cardioverter-defibrillator (Review). *Chest* 2001; 119: 1210–21.

11 Pinski S. Emergencies related to implantable cardioverter-defibrillators. *Crit Care Med* 2000; 28: N174–80.

12 Schaumann A. Managing atrial tachyarrhythmias in patients with implantable cardioverter-defibrillators. *Am J Cardiol* 1999; 83: 214D–17D.

13 Schluter T, Baum H, Plewan A *et al*. Effects of implantable cardioverter defibrillator implantation and shock application on biochemical markers of myocardial damage. *Clin Chem* 2001; 47: 459–63.

14 Weretka S, Michaelsin J, Becker R *et al*. Ventricular oversensing: a study of 101 patients implanted with dual chamber defibrillators and two different lead systems. *Pacing Clin Electrophysiol* 2003; 26: 65–70.

15 Maisel WH, Sweeney MO, Stevenson WG *et al*. Recalls and safety alerts involving pacemakers and implantable cardioverter-defibrillator generators. *JAMA* 2001; 286: 793–9.

16 Sweeney MO, Ellison KE, Shea JB *et al*. Provoked and spontaneous high-frequency, low-amplitude, respirophasic noise transients in patients with implantable cardioverter defibrillators. *J Cardiovasc Electrophsiol* 2001; 12: 402–10.

17 Glikson M, Trusty JM, Grice SK *et al*. A stepwise testing protocol for modern implantable cardioverter-defibrillator systems to prevent pacemaker-implantable cardioverter-defibrillator interactions. *Am J Cardiol* 1999; 83: 360–6.

18 Singer I. Evaluation of implantable cardioverter-defibrillator malfunction, diagnostics, and programmers, in Ellenbogen KA, Kay GN and Wilkoff BL (eds). *Clinical cardiac pacing and defibrillation*. Philadelphia: W.B. Saunders, 2000, pp. 876–94.

19 Stone K, McPherson C. Assessment and management of patients with pacemakers and implantable cardioverter defibrillators. *Crit Care Med* 2004; 32: 5155–65.

20 Hayes DL, Strathmore NF. Electromagnetic interference with implantable devices. in Ellenbogen KA, Kay GN, and Wilkoff BL (eds). *Clinical Cardiac Pacing and Defibrillation*. Philadelphia: W.B. Saunders, 2000, pp. 939–52.

21 Hayes DL, Carrillo RG, Findlay GK *et al*. State of the science: pacemaker and defibrillator interference from wireless communication devices. *Pacing Clin Electrophysiol* 1996; 19: 1419.

22 Lemon JM, Edelman S, Kirkness A. Avoidance behaviors in patients with implantable cardioverter defibrillators. *Heart Lung* 2004; 33: 176–82.

23 Dougherty C, Pyper G, Frasz H. Description of a nursing intervention program after an implantable cardioverter defibrillator. *Heart Lung* 2004; 33: 183–90.

CHAPTER 7

Pacing therapies for heart failure

Rebecca E. Lane, Martin R. Cowie, and Anthony W.C. Chow

Heart failure

Advances in the management of myocardial infarction and hypertension[1] to reduce mortality, combined with an aging population, have substantially contributed to the increasing numbers of patients with chronic heart failure. Despite optimal pharmacotherapy,[2–9] the morbidity and mortality associated with heart failure remains high. Poor quality of life and recurrent hospitalizations are common, with a 4-year survival of less than 50% (Figure 7.1).[1,10] Heart failure has now become an escalating epidemic and represents a major public health problem.

Studies have demonstrated that the frequency and mode of death is different depending on heart failure severity. In patients with mild to moderate heart failure [New York Heart Association (NYHA) Classes II and III] sudden death

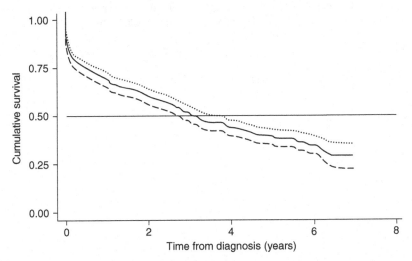

Figure 7.1 Cumulative survival of 552 incident (new) cases of heart failure identified in the London Heart Failure Studies 1995–8. Kaplan–Meier estimates with 95% pointwise confidence bands (author's own data).

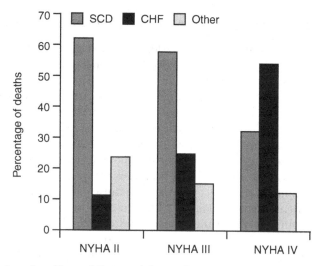

Figure 7.2 Severity of heart failure and the mode of death in the MERIT-HF study. Redrawn from the MERIT-HF Study Group. SCD sudden cardiac death, CHF congestive heart failure. *Lancet* 1999; 353: 2001–7.

is the most common mode of death, accounting for 64% and 59% deaths, respectively, and progressive heart failure causing death in 12% and 26% of patients, respectively. In contrast, in patients with more advanced heart failure (NYHA Class IV), progressive pump failure is the predominant cause of death (56% of patients), with sudden death accounting for 33% of deaths (Figure 7.2).[11]

Despite aggressive medical therapy, the prognosis for patients with advanced heart failure remains worse than many forms of cancer.[10] Until recent years, cardiac transplantation offered the only real hope for such patients, but due to the disproportionate number of potential recipients to available donors, and the extent of comorbidity in many patients, relatively few heart failure patients have qualified for or survived to transplantation.

In the last decade, device therapy has become increasingly important in the management of heart failure both in improving symptoms and for treating ventricular arrhythmias to prevent sudden death.

Biventricular pacing (BVP) or cardiac resynchronization therapy (CRT) is an adjuvant therapy for patients with symptomatic, drug refractory heart failure that has demonstrated both acute and medium-term hemodynamic benefits and functional improvements.[12–14] The implantable cardioverter-defibrillator (ICD) is highly effective at terminating life-threatening ventricular tachyarrhythmias, and in selected high-risk patients has been shown to reduce mortality.[15–18] Combined biventricular pacemakers–defibrillators may be even more effective in reducing hospitalization due to heart failure and risk of death from malignant arrhythmias.

Left bundle branch block and ventricular dyssynchrony

In normal sinus rhythm, activation of left and right ventricles occurs almost simultaneously. Left bundle branch block (LBBB) due to disease of the specialized conduction tissue within the left ventricle results in an abnormal sequence of depolarization, with significant delay of left ventricular (LV) systole and diastole compared with right ventricular activation.[19] This abnormal pattern of depolarization causes LV dyssynchrony characterized by regions of early and late ventricular contraction. It is estimated that 20–30% of patients with heart failure have LBBB on their electrocardiogram (ECG). The presence of both factors is associated with a poor prognosis.[20]

One prominent adverse effect of LBBB is to cause paradoxical movement of the interventricular septum (Figure 7.3).[21] In its most severe form, contraction of the septum occurs at the time the posterolateral LV wall is relaxing, and vice versa. The failure of simultaneous contraction of opposing LV walls results in a significant proportion of blood being shifted within the ventricular cavity instead of being ejected into the circulation. Both regional septal contraction and global ejection fraction are consequently reduced,[19] as are the peak rate of change in LV pressure (LV $\pm$ dP/dt) and cardiac output. Dyssynchronous ventricular contraction may delay both aortic and mitral valve opening, decreasing the proportion of the cardiac cycle available for LV filling and ejection, and thus further reducing stroke volume and cardiac output.[22] Normal mitral valve closure may also be affected by LBBB, which may induce or exacerbate functional mitral regurgitation.[23,24]

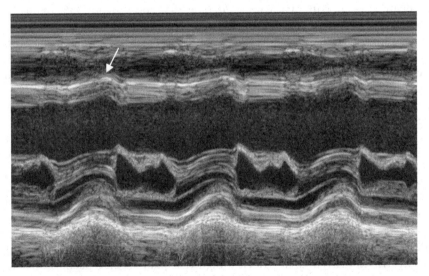

Figure 7.3 M-mode echocardiogram showing paradoxical left ventricular septal wall contraction (arrowed) and late systolic/early diastolic thickening of the posterior wall in a patient with dilated cardiomyopathy and LBBB.

In heart failure, abnormalities of ventricular conduction are frequently compounded by a prolonged PR interval resulting in additional atrioventricular (AV) dyssynchrony, which may increase the severity of mitral regurgitation.[25]

Dual chamber pacing for the treatment of heart failure

Disease of the specialized conduction tissue is common in patients with heart failure. "Conventional" permanent pacing corrects symptomatic bradycardia and may alleviate heart failure and reduce morbidity and mortality when used to treat heart block.

Animal studies suggested that an appropriately timed atrial contraction is necessary for optimal LV systolic function by increasing LV end diastolic pressure while maintaining a low left atrial pressure.[26–29] With this concept in mind, conventional dual chamber pacing (DDD) was used in the early 1990s in an attempt to improve hemodynamics in patients with drug-resistant heart failure, with emphasis on manipulation of the AV delay. A number of small studies were performed with inconsistent results.[30–34] However, retrospective analyses suggested that DDD pacing with a short AV delay may help to increase LV filling times and reduce presystolic mitral regurgitation (regurgitation through the mitral valve before the onset of mechanical systole due to elevated LV end diastolic pressure), thereby increasing cardiac output in a subgroup of patients with long PR intervals.[32,35]

It is apparent that the AV interval required to achieve optimal AV synchrony varies among individuals. In a small minority of patients right ventricular DDD pacing may provide hemodynamic benefit, but for the majority, right ventricular pacing produced no benefit or had detrimental effects on LV function. This potentially deleterious effect was evident in two large randomized controlled trials of ICDs, where a trend toward an increased incidence of new or worsened heart failure requiring hospitalization was observed in those receiving a significant amount of right ventricular pacing.[18,36] This can be explained by right ventricular pacing inducing an LBBB pattern of ventricular activation and thus exacerbating ventricular dyssynchrony and further aggravating LV dysfunction.[37]

In an attempt to provide a more physiological pattern of ventricular activation, many centers advocate right ventricular septal pacing as an alternative to right ventricular apical pacing. However, hemodynamic studies of septal pacing have also shown disparate results.[38–41]

History and hemodynamic effects of CRT

Attempts to modify or normalize electrical activation in the hope of improving mechanical function and cardiac performance led to the idea of BVP or CRT. In 1994, Cazeau and colleagues described four-chamber pacing in a patient with severe heart failure, LBBB (QRS duration 200 ms), prolonged PR interval (200 ms), and a 90 ms interatrial delay, to provide resynchronization of both atria and both ventricles. An initial acute hemodynamic study with four temporary pacing leads demonstrated an increased cardiac output from 3.9 to 5.7 L/min and decreased pulmonary capillary wedge pressure from 36 to 28 mm Hg. Following permanent implantation, the patient's functional class improved dramatically, reducing from NYHA Class IV to II.[42]

Several subsequent studies have compared the hemodynamic effects of different pacing configurations during dual chamber pacing with right ventricular or LV pacing alone and with CRT.[43–45] These demonstrated acute increases in systolic blood pressure, cardiac output, maximum LV pressure development (LV + dP/dt) and aortic pulse pressure with decreased pulmonary capillary wedge pressure during either BVP or LV pacing alone. These improvements were incremental over smaller benefits seen with right ventricular apical or septal pacing.[43,45,46]

Randomized controlled trials of CRT

In 2001, the multisite stimulation in cardiomyopathies (MUSTIC) study was published. This was a single blind, randomized, controlled crossover study in which 67 patients with severe systolic heart failure (NYHA Class III) and a wide QRS (duration >150 ms) were implanted with an atriobiventricular pacemaker. Patients were randomized to a 3-month period of inactive pacing (ventricular inhibited pacing at a basic rate of 40 bpm) and a 3-month period of active (atriobiventricular) pacing, with 48 patients completing both arms of the study. The primary endpoint was the distance walked in 6 minutes. This increased by 23% during active pacing ($p < 0.001$). The secondary endpoints, such as quality of life, hospitalizations, and peak oxygen uptake were also significantly improved.[13]

Following this, a larger Multicenter InSync Randomized Clinical Evaluation (MIRACLE) study, a double-blind randomized controlled trial was conducted. Patients were assigned to a CRT group ($n = 228$) or to a control group ($n = 225$) and followed up over a 6-month period. Inclusion criteria were moderate to severe heart failure, LV ejection fraction <35% and QRS duration >130 ms. Primary end points were NYHA functional class, quality of life, and the distance walked in 6 minutes. CRT significantly improved all of the measured endpoints as compared with the control group. Secondary endpoints, such as peak oxygen uptake, total exercise time, and ejection fraction were also significantly increased at 6 months follow-up with CRT. Hospital admissions were substantially decreased, with a 77% reduction in the total number of days hospitalized in the CRT group compared with controls, suggesting that such therapy is likely to be highly cost-effective.[12]

The Comparison of Medical Therapy, Pacing, and Defibrillation in Chronic Heart Failure (COMPANION) study was a randomized controlled trial of more than 1500 patients with ischemic or nonischemic heart failure in NYHA Class III or IV, and QRS duration >120 ms. Patients were randomised in a 1 : 2 : 2 ratio to receive optimal pharmacological therapy alone or in combination with CRT with either a pacemaker or a combined pacemaker–defibrillator. The primary composite endpoint was death or hospitalization from any cause. Similar reductions in relative risk of the primary endpoint were found in both CRT with a pacemaker (19%, $p = 0.014$) and CRT with a combined pacemaker-defibrillator (20%, $p = 0.01$) compared with medical therapy alone. CRT with a pacemaker–defibrillator significantly reduced the secondary endpoint of death from any cause by 36% ($p = 0.003$). This was the first clear demonstration of survival benefit from CRT in patients with heart failure, resulting in premature termination of the trial. CRT without a defibrillator provided a nonsignificant reduction in death from any cause by 24% ($p = 0.059$). These data have added weight to the use of combined pacemaker-defibrillator devices for improving both morbidity and mortality in selected patients.[1]

Recent reports from the CArdiac REsynchronization in Heart Failure (CARE-HF) study has further confirmed that CRT alone provides both morbidity and mortality benefits. In this trial, 813 patients were randomized to either CRT (without defibrillator) or optimal medical therapy and followed up for $2\frac{1}{2}$ years. The primary endpoints of mortality and unplanned cardiovascular hospitalization were reduced by 37% and the secondary endpoint of all cause mortality was reduced by 36% in the CRT group, again confirming the clear benefits of CRT in treating selected patients with heart failure.[47]

Current indications for CRT

The current (updated in 2002) American Heart Association guidelines for indications for CRT provided a Class IIa indication (evidence obtained from at least one well-designed controlled study without randomization) with level of evidence A (at least one randomized controlled trial as part of a body of literature of overall good quality and consistency addressing the specific recommendation).[48] Patients deemed suitable for such therapy are those with refractory symptomatic heart failure despite optimal medical therapy (NYHA Class III or IV) with idiopathic or ischemic dilated cardiomyopathy (LV end-diastolic diameter >55 mm), a prolonged QRS interval (>130 ms), and a poorly functioning left ventricle (LV ejection fraction <35%).

The majority of randomized controlled trials have included only patients in sinus rhythm, but there is a growing body of evidence demonstrating symptomatic and functional benefit in patients with chronic atrial fibrillation and LBBB.[49–51] Similarly, while most trials have studied patients with LBBB, patients with right bundle branch block (RBBB) and nonspecific intraventricular delay may also improve following CRT, but this remains to be fully substantiated.[52]

Chronic right ventricular pacing for conventional bradycardiac indications induces ventricular dyssynchrony and may exacerbate heart failure. In those patients with preexisting LV impairment, CRT should be considered from the outset. Following pacing, vigilance for the development of, or deterioration in heart failure is important. In this situation, upgrading dual chamber devices to provide CRT has been shown in small observational studies to improve LV function and symptoms.[51,53]

Patient selection

Until recently, a broad QRS duration has formed the main criterion for selecting patients as candidates for CRT. However, QRS duration provides only an indirect measure of ventricular dyssynchrony with only moderate sensitivity and specificity. In large randomized controlled trials of CRT that used traditional ECG criteria (LBBB, QRS duration >120 ms) for inclusion, ~20–30% patients failed to respond clinically.[12,54,55] Furthermore, 30–40% of heart failure patients with abnormal QRS duration >120 ms do not exhibit LV dyssynchrony, which may account for the lack of response to CRT. Conversely, ~25% of patients with heart failure and a narrow QRS have significant LV dyssynchrony, and as such may benefit from CRT, but previously would have been excluded.[56] Not surprisingly, CRT has been proven to be of benefit in selected patients with a narrow QRS duration and evidence of ventricular dyssynchrony.[57]

In an attempt to improve patient selection and predict clinical response to CRT, other noninvasive tests have been increasingly used to assess dyssynchrony.[58,59] Although cardiac magnetic resonance imaging (MRI) can be used, most emphasis has focused on echocardiographically guided techniques, in particular tissue Doppler imaging,[60] because of its widespread availability, lower cost, and reproducibility.

Use of echocardiography to guide patient selection for CRT
Some of the most commonly used echocardiographic parameters are described below.

AV dyssynchrony
Atrioventricular dyssynchrony may occur as a consequence of ventricular dyssynchrony or due to a prolonged PR interval,[61] and can result in impaired LV filling. An LV filling time (time from onset of the E wave to the end of the A wave on transmitral pulsed wave Doppler) of < 40% cardiac cycle (or R–R interval on the ECG) is suggestive of AV dyssynchrony.[61]

Inter- and intraventricular dyssynchrony
Much of the benefits observed following CRT are related to improved synchrony of contraction *within* the left ventricle. Incoordination within the left ventricle or intraventricular dyssynchrony should therefore be distinguished from interventricular dyssynchrony, which implies a delay between right and left ventricular contraction.

A prolonged aortic preejection time (>140 ms) measured as the time from QRS onset on the ECG (electrical activation of the heart) to the start of Doppler flow in the aortic outflow tract (mechanical force generating flow in the

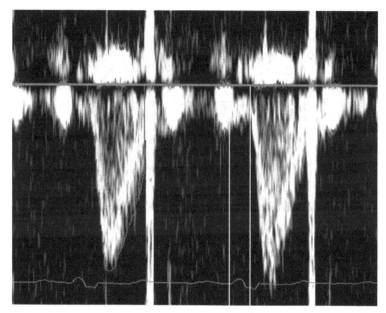

Figure 7.4 Pulsed Doppler measured in the aortic outflow tract with simultaneous ECG recording. Time between vertical lines represents the aortic preejection time. Tracing around the Doppler envelope the aortic velocity time integral may be calculated and used to optimize pacemaker programming postimplant.

aorta) is considered a marker of intraventricular dyssynchrony (Figure 7.4).[61] The difference between aortic and pulmonary preejection times provides a measure of interventricular dyssynchrony and is considered abnormal when >40 ms.[61]

Using either M-mode echocardiography or tissue Doppler imaging, delays in LV segmental longitudinal contraction can be demonstrated.[61] Tissue Doppler imaging has now been used extensively to study both inter and intraventricular dyssynchrony,[62,63] and may be useful in predicting short-term efficacy of CRT (Figure 7.5).[64]

The first prospective study of CRT with patient selection based on mechanical as opposed to electrical criteria reported clinical improvement in 85% of patients.[61] Inclusion criteria for device implantation were measurements of dyssynchrony calculated from standard pulsed Doppler and M-mode techniques.

In another study, the presence of combined intra- and interventricular dyssynchrony, as measured by pulsed wave tissue Doppler imaging, were found to be the best predictors of LV functional recovery and reverse remodeling after CRT, while QRS duration was of no value.[65] It seems likely therefore that patient selection based on echocardiographic assessment will supersede the ECG.

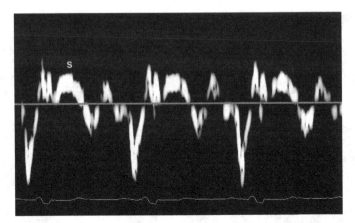

Figure 7.5 Pulsed wave tissue Doppler imaging of the basal septum. The S wave represents longitudinal shortening toward the transducer at the cardiac apex. Regional electromechanical delay may be measured from the start of the QRS complex on the ECG to the onset or the peak of the S wave. Regional differences in electromechanical delay are used to calculate inter- and intra-ventricular dyssynchrony.

Device implantation

An epicardial approach was first used to pace the left ventricle.[66,67] This required a limited thoracotomy or thoracoscopy under general anesthesia, which in elderly frail patients incurs significant operative risk. This open surgical approach, however, has the distinct advantage of facilitating LV stimulation from any epicardial site and hence optimal lead placement. LV thresholds are, however, frequently raised and delayed exit block and associated loss of LV capture have been reported.

This approach has now been replaced largely by a fully transvenous approach first reported by Daubert and colleagues in 1998, using the venous drainage system of the heart to gain access to the left ventricle.[68] This technique involves passage of a pacing lead from the right atrium into the coronary sinus, finally positioning the pacing lead into a venous tributary overlying the LV free wall (Figure 7.6).

Using a subclavian vein puncture, specially shaped guide catheters and guidewires are used to cannulate the coronary sinus, which is often difficult in patients with dilated hearts and distorted anatomy (Figure 7.7). To delineate the coronary venous anatomy and help select a target vein, a veno-occlusive balloon may be used to assist in performing a coronary sinus venogram (Figures 7.8 and 7.9).

Many coronary sinus pacing leads and wires of different shapes and stiffness have been designed to gain access to small and often tortuous venous tributaries. Traditional over-the-wire angioplasty techniques have been increasingly used with the development of side-wire[69] and fully over-the-wire leads (Figure 7.10a and b).[70] Advances in pacing lead technology and left heart

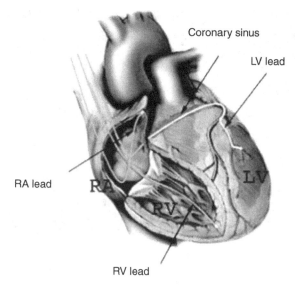

Figure 7.6 Diagram of lead placement during BVP. The RA lead is positioned within the RA appendage. The RV lead passes from the right atrium across the tricuspid valve and is positioned at the RV apex. The LV lead passes from the right atrium into the coronary sinus. It is advanced until the tip of the lead is within a lateral vein overlying the lateral wall of the left ventricle.

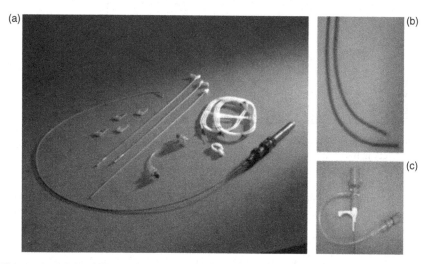

Figure 7.7 (a) LV delivery system including guide catheters through which a steerable catheter may be inserted to facilitate coronary sinus access. (b) Preshaped guide catheters to intubate the coronary sinus. (c) Hemostatic valve connected to the end of the guide catheter.

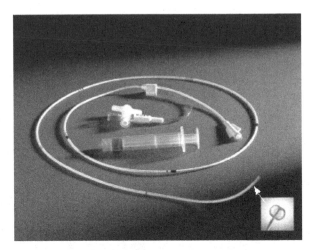

Figure 7.8 Veno-occlusive balloon catheter. Insert: the inflated balloon at the catheter tip designed to occlude the coronary sinus. Contrast is injected down the side port through the central lumen of the catheter to perform a coronary sinus venogram.

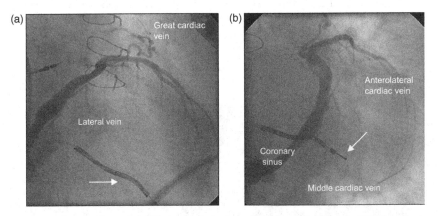

Figure 7.9 Venograms performed in a patient undergoing upgrade of an ICD to a biventricular ICD. The ICD lead can be seen already positioned in the RV apex (arrowed). Venograms are performed using different projections–(a) right anterior oblique, and (b) left anterior oblique. A small lateral vein can be seen. A larger anterolateral vein can be seen overlying the lateral free wall and collateralizing with the middle cardiac vein along the inferior wall of the left ventricle.

delivery systems have simplified the procedure and dramatically increased implant success rate to between 82% and 92%.[68,71–73] CRT implants remain highly complex and require considerable skill and experience to achieve success.

Left ventricular endocardial pacing using a transeptal approach has also been described, but concerns regarding the potential thromboembolic risk

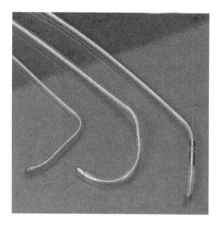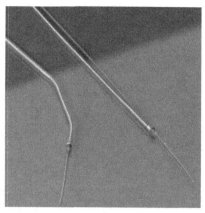

Figure 7.10 LV leads. (a) Different preshaped left ventricular leads. (b) Over-the-wire lead and side-wire lead.

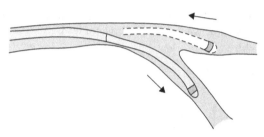

Figure 7.11 Preshaped LV lead. The lead tip is advanced to just past the bifurcation. On withdrawal of the stylet the pacing lead returns to its preshaped state and the tip falls into the target vein.

and the need for anticoagulation both at the time of implantation and long-term have limited its wider application.[74–76] LV epicardial pacing remains an option where transvenous pacing has failed or is precluded.

Pacing sites

There remains considerable debate about the optimal pacing sites for CRT.

Preliminary evidence suggests that optimal improvements in LV performance may be achieved by pacing the left ventricle at the latest site of contraction.[77] Although improvements in cardiac function and exercise capacity have also been reported following CRT regardless of pacing site,[78] preimplant assessment with tissue Doppler imaging or MRI may be useful in identifying the latest sites of LV contraction to guide LV lead placement.[59,77,79] The lateral free wall typically shows delayed contraction in patients with LBBB and is the most common target for LV pacing. It is also generally accepted that pacing scarred akinetic regions should be avoided. In practice, the choice of LV

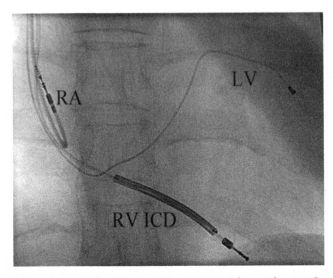

Figure 7.12 Fluoroscopy of final lead positions. (RA – right atrial active fixation lead. RVICD – right ventricular active fixation defibrillator lead. LV – left ventricular passive fixation lead.)

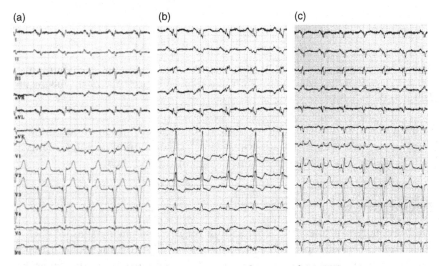

Figure 7.13 Twelve lead ECGs showing (a) RV, (b) LV, and (c) BVP.

pacing site at implantation is frequently determined by individual coronary venous anatomy. The coronary venous system is often highly collateralized allowing the use of different veins to reach the same target area (Figure 7.9). Fluoroscopy or chest X-ray to document final lead positions is recommended (Figure 7.12).

Testing and technical aspects

During implantation, 12 lead ECGs are recorded to ensure capture (Figure 7.13). Standard lead testing is performed to determine pacing thresholds, sensing, impedance, and stability. Higher LV thresholds are common, with 4 V generally being the ideal upper limit, though higher thresholds can be accepted if no alternative sites are found. Often small adjustments in LV tip position can provide substantial changes in pacing parameters. Until recently, most LV leads have been unipolar leads and pacing has been from right ventricular ring to LV tip. Testing using this configuration is therefore recommended during implantation. Phrenic nerve or diaphragmatic stimulation is a commonly encountered problem with CRT and careful testing to avoid this phenomenon is essential at implantation since lead repositioning may be required.

Device selection

It has been suggested that in patients with advanced heart failure CRT simply changes the mode of death from one of progressive heart failure to sudden death. Indications for implantable defibrillators continue to expand within the heart failure population.[18,80–82] Consequently, when implanting a biventricular pacemaker the decision whether to implant a combined pacemaker-ICD has become increasingly complex. In the Companion study, a statistically significant mortality benefit was only found among those patients receiving a combined device, though other studies such as CARE-HF suggest CRT itself reduces mortality. Refinement of the risk stratification for sudden cardiac death among patients with heart failure is likely to be crucial in guiding appropriate device selection to enable a safe, cost-effective practice.

Implantable cardioverter defibrillator trials have further influenced the use of CRT since right ventricular pacing has been shown to cause worsening heart failure.[18,36] For patients with heart failure and bradycardia or heart block, conventional right ventricular pacing may exacerbate LV dysfunction. In such instances, implanting a CRT device may be the ideal option.

When implanting a biventricular pacemaker ±ICD stringent testing is essential to ensure acceptable defibrillator thresholds. In patients with severely dilated ventricles the use of active fixation ICD leads and high-output devices should be given consideration.

Acute complications and trouble-shooting

Complications include those of conventional pacing such as periprocedural bleeding, pneumothorax, and arm edema due to venous occlusion.

Commonly encountered acute complications associated with CRT are predominantly related to LV lead placement. Inability to deploy the LV lead accounts for most of the 8% reported implant failure.[12] This may be due to inability to cannulate the coronary sinus, coronary sinus dissection or perforation, or unacceptable LV pacing parameters. Coronary sinus trauma is seldom associated with any clinical sequelae, but may rarely require pericardiocentesis.[12,83] Valves or strictures within the coronary sinus may further hamper LV lead deployment. Poor thresholds may occur around areas of myocardial scar while achieving lead stability may be problematic with recurrent LV lead displacement. Diaphragmatic pacing at relatively low outputs may also preclude the use of certain LV pacing sites.

Implantation requires patients to lie flat and careful preparation is essential to ensure a euvolaemic state, minimizing the risk of periprocedural pulmonary edema. Conversely, excessive diuresis and volume depletion will risk hypotension and potentiate the risk of contrast-induced nephropathy.

Chronic complications and trouble-shooting

Left ventricular lead displacement is most common in the first few weeks but may occur up to 1 year after implantation. This may be associated with loss of LV capture and hence CRT, with patients reporting worsening of heart failure symptoms. "Micro" left ventricular displacements may also precipitate problems with phrenic nerve stimulation. Newer devices now possess independently programmable left and right ventricular outputs and sensing configurations [left ventricular tip (cathode) to right ventricular ring (anode), left ventricular tip to right ventricular coil, left ventricular tip to ring, left ventricular ring to tip]. If device reprogramming fails, lead repositioning is required.

Device-related complications are unusual, but inappropriate interactions can occur. AV crosstalk is a potential problem during CRT and usually occurs where atrial sensing occurs on an LV lead implanted in the great cardiac vein, with the potential to cause ventricular standstill in pacemaker-dependent patients. Where this cannot be avoided, a right ventricular-only sensing configuration should be programmed.[84]

There remains debate about the potential proarrhythmic or antiarrhythmic effects of CRT. The frequency and duration of ventricular ectopics and arrhythmias have been shown to be significantly reduced,[85–87] but proarrhythmia with LV stimulation has also been reported.[88] Malignant ventricular arrhythmias are common among patients with heart failure.[89,90] and combined biventricular pacemaker-defibrillators are increasingly being implanted to offer additional protection from sudden cardiac death.

Paroxysmal or persistent atrial fibrillation is also common among heart failure patients who frequently have dilated atria with significant mitral regurgitation. Atrial arrhythmias may similarly be detected at follow-up by CRT device interrogation and may alert the need for adjustment of pharmacotherapy (additional antiarrhythmics and anticoagulation). There are also reports that CRT can reduce atrial fibrillation or restore sinus rhythm with improvement in LV function. In cases of persistent atrial fibrillation the device should be reprogrammed to biventricular VVI mode.

Inappropriate shocks have occurred in some combined biventricular pacemaker-defibrillator devices caused by rapid ventricular rates or double counting of ventricular events in a detection algorithm that senses from both right and left ventricular leads.[91,92] To minimize this possibility, tachycardia therapy decisions in newer ICDs determine the cycle length by using right ventricular sensed events only.

Pacemaker infections are always serious and usually necessitate removal of the entire system. Prophylactic intravenous antibiotics should be given preimplantation and an oral course subsequently completed. To date there is only limited experience of coronary sinus lead extraction,[93] but with increasing numbers of devices being implanted this will inevitably grow.

Postimplant follow-up

The aim of CRT in heart failure is to reduce mechanical dyssynchrony, thereby enabling the heart to contract more efficiently, increasing LV ejection fraction and cardiac output, but with less work and lower oxygen consumption.[94] Following CRT, two-dimensional and Doppler echocardiography, tissue Doppler imaging and three-dimensional reconstruction may be helpful to monitor "reverse" remodeling of the LV and reduced ventricular dyssynchrony.[64,95–98] Predischarge pacing and ICD checks should be standard practice to accurately record pacing parameters and to optimize device function. Echocardiographic-guided programming of AV and interventricular delays is essential for ensuring maximal benefit from CRT.

AV optimization

Optimization of the AV delay following pacing has traditionally been achieved using Doppler echocardiography to maximize LV filling time and minimize presystolic mitral regurgitation (Figure 7.14).[99]

Interventricular delay optimization

In more advanced biventricular pacemakers it is now possible to alter the interventricular delay, to allow either left or right ventricular preactivation. Evidence now suggests that in many patients, optimal hemodynamic benefits are observed with sequential CRT. Echocardiography, such as measurement of the maximal aortic velocity time integral ("stroke distance") may be used to guide programming of the interventricular delay postimplantation (Figure 7.4).[100–102]

Hemodynamic and clinical response to CRT can occur very rapidly (within minutes to hours). Postimplantation follow-up must focus on vigilance for potential complications and optimization of clinical response.

Concurrent adjustment of medication is essential to derive optimal benefit from CRT. Antianginal therapy may need to be adjusted as patients with a good response to CRT will increase exercise capacity because they are no longer limited by severe LV dysfunction and may develop anginal symptoms.

Enhanced cardiac output might increase renal perfusion to promote diuresis resulting in volume depletion and hypotension. A combination of improved

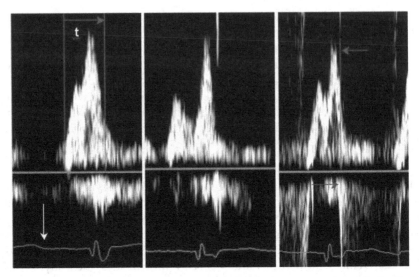

Figure 7.14 Optimization of AV delay. LV inflow pulsed wave Doppler at the level of mitral valve leaflets. (a) AV delay 160 ms: Uniphasic transmitral flow (fused E and A wave) with reduced LV filling time (t) < 40% R–R interval. The onset of filling is delayed commencing after the end of the T wave on the ECG (white arrow). (b) AV delay 90 ms: Mitral valve closure line coincides with the end of the A wave maximizing LV filling time and restoring biphasic transmitral flow with E- and A-wave separation. (c) AV delay 70 ms: The end of the A wave is now truncated by mitral valve closure (seen arrowed and aliasing), with the commencement of mitral regurgitation and reduced LV filling time. AV optimization can now be improved by increasing the AV delay in 10 ms increments until mitral valve closure line coincides with the end of the A wave without truncation.

symptoms and increased diuresis means that diuretic requirements are frequently reduced. CRT may increase blood pressure while preventing bradycardia and may therefore facilitate safe increments in β-blockers and angiotensin converting enzyme inhibitors or angiotensin receptor blockers. Devices that measure thoracic impedance to provide continuous hemodynamic monitoring are being developed and may in the future be used to guide fine adjustments of pharmacotherapy.

Univentricular LV pacing

Several short-term studies have demonstrated similar hemodynamic improvements from univentricular LV pacing compared with BVP.[43-45] One-year follow-up of patients paced exclusively from the left ventricle showed significant improvements in NYHA class, 6-minutes' walk distance, peak oxygen uptake, LV end-diastolic diameter and mitral regurgitation.[103] However, long-term studies on this pacing mode are still lacking.

Conclusion

There is now a substantial body of evidence to show that CRT with BVP provides clear symptomatic benefits in selected patients with heart failure and ventricular dyssynchrony. CRT must be used as adjuvant therapy and not as an alternative to optimal medical treatment. The potential indications for CRT are likely to expand; but the process of patient selection needs further refinement to ensure that only individuals who will benefit are offered this therapy. Careful device selection, implantation, and programming are essential for minimizing procedural complications and maximizing patient response. Echocardiography and tissue Doppler imaging are likely to be key factors for optimizing these processes.

There is accumulating evidence for the wider application of combined CRT–ICDs in patients with LV dysfunction. Recent trial data suggest that CRT alone confers a mortality benefit, but whether additional ICD backup improves survival further remains to be clarified by ongoing randomized trials. The role of device therapy for heart failure is set to expand with inevitable cost implications. A multidisciplinary approach of primary care physicians and specialists in heart failure, electrophysiology, and echocardiography will ensure the most effective implementation of this developing therapy.

References

1 Cowie MR, Wood DA, Coats AJ et al. Incidence and aetiology of heart failure; a population-based study. *Eur Heart J* 1999; 20: 421–8.
2 Effect of enalapril on survival in patients with reduced left ventricular ejection fractions and congestive heart failure. The SOLVD Investigators. *N Engl J Med* 1991; 325: 293–302.
3 Effect of enalapril on mortality and the development of heart failure in asymptomatic patients with reduced left ventricular ejection fractions. The SOLVD Investigators. *N Engl J Med* 1992; 327: 685–91.
4 Kjekshus J, Swedberg K, Snapinn S. Effects of enalapril on long-term mortality in severe congestive heart failure. CONSENSUS Trial Group. *Am J Cardiol* 1992; 69: 103–7.
5 Pitt B, Zannad F, Remme WJ et al. The effect of spironolactone on morbidity and mortality in patients with severe heart failure. Randomized Aldactone Evaluation Study Investigators. *N Engl J Med* 1999; 341: 709–17.
6 Hjalmarson A, Goldstein S, Fagerberg B et al. Effects of controlled-release metoprolol on total mortality, hospitalizations, and well-being in patients with heart failure: the Metoprolol CR/XL Randomized Intervention Trial in congestive heart failure (MERIT-HF). MERIT-HF Study Group. *JAMA* 2000; 283: 1295–302.
7 Packer M, Bristow MR, Cohn JN et al. The effect of carvedilol on morbidity and mortality in patients with chronic heart failure. U.S. Carvedilol Heart Failure Study Group. *N Engl J Med* 1996; 334: 1349–55.

8 Packer M, Fowler MB, Roecker EB *et al.* Effect of carvedilol on the morbidity of patients with severe chronic heart failure: results of the carvedilol prospective randomized cumulative survival (COPERNICUS) study. *Circulation* 2002; 106: 2194–9.

9 Konstam MA, Rousseau MF, Kronenberg MW *et al.* Effects of the angiotensin converting enzyme inhibitor enalapril on the long-term progression of left ventricular dysfunction in patients with heart failure. The SOLVD Investigators. *Circulation* 1992; 86: 431–8.

10 Stewart S, MacIntyre K, Hole DJ, Capewell S, McMurray JJ. More "malignant" than cancer? Five-year survival following a first admission for heart failure. *Eur J Heart Fail* 2001; 3: 315–22.

11 Effect of metoprolol CR/XL in chronic heart failure: Metoprolol CR/XL Randomised Intervention Trial in Congestive Heart Failure (MERIT-HF). *Lancet* 1999; 353: 2001–7.

12 Abraham WT, Fisher WG, Smith AL *et al.* Cardiac resynchronization in chronic heart failure. *N Engl J Med* 2002; 346: 1845–53.

13 Cazeau S, Leclercq C, Lavergne T *et al.* Effects of multisite biventricular pacing in patients with heart failure and intraventricular conduction delay. *N Engl J Med* 2001; 344: 873–80.

14 Huth C, Friedl A, Klein H, Auricchio A. Pacing therapies for congestive heart failure considering the results of the PATH-CHF study. *Z Kardiol* 2001; 90: 10–15.

15 A comparison of antiarrhythmic-drug therapy with implantable defibrillators in patients resuscitated from near-fatal ventricular arrhythmias. The Antiarrhythmics versus Implantable Defibrillators (AVID) Investigators. *N Engl J Med* 1997; 337: 1576–83.

16 Connolly SJ, Hallstrom AP, Cappato R *et al.* Meta-analysis of the implantable cardioverter defibrillator secondary prevention trials. AVID, CASH and CIDS studies. Antiarrhythmics vs Implantable Defibrillator study. Cardiac Arrest Study Hamburg. Canadian Implantable Defibrillator Study. *Eur Heart J* 2000; 21: 2071–8.

17 Buxton AE, Lee KL, Fisher JD *et al.* A randomized study of the prevention of sudden death in patients with coronary artery disease. Multicenter Unsustained Tachycardia Trial Investigators. *N Engl J Med* 1999; 341: 1882–90.

18 Moss AJ, Zareba W, Hall WJ *et al.* Prophylactic implantation of a defibrillator in patients with myocardial infarction and reduced ejection fraction. *N Engl J Med* 2002; 346: 877–83.

19 Grines CL, Bashore TM, Boudoulas H *et al.* Functional abnormalities in isolated left bundle branch block. The effect of interventricular asynchrony. *Circulation* 1989; 79: 845–53.

20 Baldasseroni S, Opasich C, Gorini M *et al.* Left bundle-branch block is associated with increased 1-year sudden and total mortality rate in 5517 outpatients with congestive heart failure: a report from the Italian network on congestive heart failure. *Am Heart J* 2002; 143: 398–405.

21 Zoneraich S, Zoneraich O, Rhee JJ. Echocardiographic evaluation of septal motion in patients with artificial pacemakers: vectorcardiographic correlations. *Am Heart J* 1977; 93: 596–602.

22 Zhou Q, Henein M, Coats A, Gibson D. Different effects of abnormal activation and myocardial disease on left ventricular ejection and filling times. *Heart* 2000; 84: 272–6.

23 Xiao HB, Lee CH, Gibson DG. Effect of left bundle branch block on diastolic function in dilated cardiomyopathy. *Br Heart J* 1991; 66: 443–7.

24 Breithardt OA, Sinha AM, Schwammenthal E *et al.* Acute effects of cardiac resynchronization therapy on functional mitral regurgitation in advanced systolic heart failure. *J Am Coll Cardiol* 2003; 41: 765–70.

25 Ishikawa T, Sumita S, Kimura K *et al.* Efficacy of atrioventricular sequential pacing and diastolic mitral regurgitation in patients with intrinsic atrioventricular conduction. *Jpn Circ J* 2000; 64: 579–82.

26 Jochim K. The conrtibution of the auricles to ventricular filling in complete heart block. *Am J Physiol* 1938; 122: 639–45.

27 Gessel RA. Auricular systole and its relation to ventricular output. *Am J Physiol* 1911; 29: 32–63.

28 Mitchell JH, Gilmore JP, Sarnoff SJ. The transport function of the atrium: factors influencing the relation between mean left atrial pressure and left ventricular end diastolic pressure. *Am J Cardiol* 1962; 9: 237–47.

29 Skinner NS Jr, Mitchell JH, Wallace AJ, Sarnoff SJ. Haemodynamic effects of altering the timing of atrial systole. *Am J Physiol* 1963; 205: 499–503.

30 Hochleitner M, Hortnagl H, Ng CK *et al.* Usefulness of physiologic dual-chamber pacing in drug-resistant idiopathic dilated cardiomyopathy. *Am J Cardiol* 1990; 66: 198–202.

31 Linde C, Gadler F, Edner M *et al.* Results of atrioventricular synchronous pacing with optimized delay in patients with severe congestive heart failure. *Am J Cardiol* 1995; 75: 919–23.

32 Brecker SJ, Xiao HB, Sparrow J *et al.* Effects of dual-chamber pacing with short atrioventricular delay in dilated cardiomyopathy. *Lancet* 1992; 340: 1308–12.

33 Gold MR, Feliciano Z, Gottlieb SS *et al.* Dual-chamber pacing with a short atrioventricular delay in congestive heart failure: a randomized study. *J Am Coll Cardiol* 1995; 26: 967–73.

34 Innes D, Leitch JW, Fletcher PJ. VDD pacing at short atrioventricular intervals does not improve cardiac output in patients with dilated heart failure. *Pacing Clin Electrophysiol* 1994; 17: 959–65.

35 Nishimura RA, Hayes DL, Holmes DR, Jr. *et al.* Mechanism of hemodynamic improvement by dual-chamber pacing for severe left ventricular dysfunction: an acute Doppler and catheterization hemodynamic study. *J Am Coll Cardiol* 1995; 25: 281–8.

36 Wilkoff BL, Cook JR, Epstein AE *et al.* Dual-chamber pacing or ventricular backup pacing in patients with an implantable defibrillator: the Dual Chamber and VVI Implantable Defibrillator (DAVID) Trial. *JAMA* 2002; 288: 3115–23.

37 Prinzen FW, Hunter WC, Wyman BT *et al.* Mapping of regional myocardial strain and work during ventricular pacing: experimental study using magnetic resonance imaging tagging. *J Am Coll Cardiol* 1999; 33: 1735–42.

38 Cowell R, Morris-Thurgood J, Ilsley C *et al.* Septal short atrioventricular delay pacing: additional hemodynamic improvements in heart failure. *Pacing Clin Electrophysiol* 1994; 17: 1980–3.

39 Gold MR, Shorofsky SR, Metcalf MD *et al.* The acute hemodynamic effects of right ventricular septal pacing in patients with congestive heart failure secondary to ischemic or idiopathic dilated cardiomyopathy. *Am J Cardiol* 1997; 79: 679–81.

40 Rosenqvist M, Bergfeldt L, Haga Y *et al.* The effect of ventricular activation sequence on cardiac performance during pacing. *Pacing Clin Electrophysiol* 1996; 19: 1279–86.

41 Takagi Y, Dumpis Y, Usui A *et al.* Effects of proximal ventricular septal pacing on hemodynamics and ventricular activation. *Pacing Clin Electrophysiol* 1999; 22: 1777–81.

42 Cazeau S, Ritter P, Bakdach S *et al.* Four chamber pacing in dilated cardiomyopathy. *Pacing Clin Electrophysiol* 1994; 17: 1974–9.

43 Blanc JJ, Etienne Y, Gilard M *et al.* Evaluation of different ventricular pacing sites in patients with severe heart failure: results of an acute hemodynamic study. *Circulation* 1997; 96: 3273–7.

44 Kass DA, Chen CH, Curry C *et al.* Improved left ventricular mechanics from acute VDD pacing in patients with dilated cardiomyopathy and ventricular conduction delay. *Circulation* 1999; 99: 1567–73.

45 Leclercq C, Cazeau S, Le Breton H *et al.* Acute hemodynamic effects of biventricular DDD pacing in patients with end-stage heart failure. *J Am Coll Cardiol* 1998; 32: 1825–31.

46 Auricchio A, Stellbrink C, Block M *et al.* Effect of pacing chamber and atrioventricular delay on acute systolic function of paced patients with congestive heart failure. The Pacing Therapies for Congestive Heart Failure Study Group. The Guidant Congestive Heart Failure Research Group. *Circulation* 1999; 99: 2993–3001.

47 Cleland JG, Daubert JC, Erdmann E *et al.* The effect of cardiac resynchronization on morbidity and mortality in heart failure. *N Engl J Med* 2005; 352: 1539–49.

48 Gregoratos G, Abrams J, Epstein AE *et al.* ACC/AHA/NASPE 2002 guideline update for implantation of cardiac pacemakers and antiarrhythmia devices: summary article: a report of the American College of Cardiology/American Heart Association Task Force on Practice Guidelines (ACC/AHA/NASPE Committee to Update the 1998 Pacemaker Guidelines). *Circulation* 2002; 106: 2145–61.

49 Leclercq C, Victor F, Alonso C *et al.* Comparative effects of permanent biventricular pacing for refractory heart failure in patients with stable sinus rhythm or chronic atrial fibrillation. *Am J Cardiol* 2000; 85: 1154–6, A9.

50 Leclercq C, Walker S, Linde C *et al.* Comparative effects of permanent biventricular and right-univentricular pacing in heart failure patients with chronic atrial fibrillation. *Eur Heart J* 2002; 23: 1780–7.

51 Leon AR, Greenberg JM, Kanuru N *et al.* Cardiac resynchronization in patients with congestive heart failure and chronic atrial fibrillation: effect of upgrading to biventricular pacing after chronic right ventricular pacing. *J Am Coll Cardiol* 2002; 39: 1258–63.

52 Garrigue S, Reuter S, Labeque JN *et al.* Usefulness of biventricular pacing in patients with congestive heart failure and right bundle branch block. *Am J Cardiol* 2001; 88: 1436–41, A8.

53 Baker CM, Christopher TJ, Smith PF *et al.* Addition of a left ventricular lead to conventional pacing systems in patients with congestive heart failure: feasibility, safety, and early results in 60 consecutive patients. *Pacing Clin Electrophysiol* 2002; 25: 1166–71.

54 Bax JJ, Marwick TH, Molhoek SG *et al.* Left ventricular dyssynchrony predicts benefit of cardiac resynchronization therapy in patients with end-stage heart failure before pacemaker implantation. *Am J Cardiol* 2003; 92: 1238–40.

55 Molhoek SG, Bax JJ, van Erven L *et al.* Effectiveness of resynchronization therapy in patients with end-stage heart failure. *Am J Cardiol* 2002; 90: 379–83.

56 Bleeker GB, Schalij MJ, Molhoek SG *et al.* Relationship between QRS duration and left ventricular dyssynchrony in patients with end-stage heart failure. *J Cardiovasc Electrophysiol* 2004; 15: 544–9.

57 Gasparini M, Mantica M, Galimberti P *et al.* Beneficial effects of biventricular pacing in patients with a "narrow" QRS. *Pacing Clin Electrophysiol* 2003; 26: 169–74.

58 O'Dell WG, McCulloch AD. Imaging three-dimensional cardiac function. *Annu Rev Biomed Eng* 2000; 2: 431–56.

59 Nelson GS, Curry CW, Wyman BT *et al.* Predictors of systolic augmentation from left ventricular preexcitation in patients with dilated cardiomyopathy and intraventricular conduction delay. *Circulation* 2000; 101: 2703–9.

60 Yu CM, Fung WH, Lin H *et al.* Predictors of left ventricular reverse remodeling after cardiac resynchronization therapy for heart failure secondary to idiopathic dilated or ischemic cardiomyopathy. *Am J Cardiol* 2003; 91: 684–8.

61 Cazeau S, Bordachar P, Jauvert G *et al.* Echocardiographic modeling of cardiac dyssynchrony before and during multisite stimulation: a prospective study. *Pacing Clin Electrophysiol* 2003; 26: 137–43.

62 Garrigue S, Jais P, Espil G *et al.* Comparison of chronic biventricular pacing between epicardial and endocardial left ventricular stimulation using Doppler tissue imaging in patients with heart failure. *Am J Cardiol* 2001; 88: 858–62.

63 Pitzalis MV, Iacoviello M, Romito R *et al.* Cardiac resynchronization therapy tailored by echocardiographic evaluation of ventricular asynchrony. *J Am Coll Cardiol* 2002; 40: 1615–22.

64 Sogaard P, Kim WY, Jensen HK *et al.* Impact of acute biventricular pacing on left ventricular performance and volumes in patients with severe heart failure. A tissue doppler and three-dimensional echocardiographic study. *Cardiology* 2001; 95: 173–82.

65 Penicka M, Bartunek J, De Bruyne B *et al.* Improvement of left ventricular function after cardiac resynchronization therapy is predicted by tissue Doppler Imaging echocardiography. *Circulation* 2004; 109: 978–83.

66 Auricchio A, Stellbrink C, Sack S *et al.* The Pacing Therapies for Congestive Heart Failure (PATH-CHF) study: rationale, design, and endpoints of a prospective randomized multicenter study. *Am J Cardiol* 1999; 83: 130D–5D.

67 Cazeau S, Ritter P, Lazarus A *et al.* Multisite pacing for end-stage heart failure: early experience. *Pacing Clin Electrophysiol* 1996; 19: 1748–57.

68 Daubert JC, Ritter P, Le Breton H *et al.* Permanent left ventricular pacing with transvenous leads inserted into the coronary veins. *Pacing Clin Electrophysiol* 1998; 21: 239–45.

69 Walker S, Levy T, Rex S *et al.* The use of a "side-wire" permanent transvenous pacing electrode for left ventricular pacing. *Europace* 1999; 1: 197–200.

70 Yu CM, Miu R. A new technique for the transvenous implantation of the over-the-wire left ventricular pacing lead in a patient with heart failure. *J Interv Card Electrophysiol* 2002; 7: 189–91.

71 Purerfellner H, Nesser HJ, Winter S *et al.* Transvenous left ventricular lead implantation with the EASYTRAK lead system: the European experience. *Am J Cardiol* 2000; 86: K157–64.

72 Auricchio A, Klein H, Tockman B *et al*. Transvenous biventricular pacing for heart failure: can the obstacles be overcome? *Am J Cardiol* 1999; 83: 136D–42D.

73 Gras D, Mabo P, Tang T *et al*. Multisite pacing as a supplemental treatment of congestive heart failure: preliminary results of the Medtronic Inc. InSync Study. *Pacing Clin Electrophysiol* 1998; 21: 2249–55.

74 Jais P, Douard H, Shah DC *et al*. Endocardial biventricular pacing. *Pacing Clin Electrophysiol* 1998; 21: 2128–31.

75 Jais P, Takahashi A, Garrigue S *et al*. Mid-term follow-up of endocardial biventricular pacing. *Pacing Clin Electrophysiol* 2000; 23: 1744–7.

76 Leclercq F, Hager FX, Macia JC *et al*. Left ventricular lead insertion using a modified transseptal catheterization technique: a totally endocardial approach for permanent biventricular pacing in end-stage heart failure. *Pacing Clin Electrophysiol* 1999; 22: 1570–5.

77 Ansalone G, Giannantoni P, Ricci R *et al*. Doppler myocardial imaging to evaluate the effectiveness of pacing sites in patients receiving biventricular pacing. *J Am Coll Cardiol* 2002; 39: 489–99.

78 Gasparini M, Mantica M, Galimberti P *et al*. Is the left ventricular lateral wall the best lead implantation site for cardiac resynchronization therapy? *Pacing Clin Electrophysiol* 2003; 26: 162–8.

79 Bax JJ, Ansalone G, Breithardt OA *et al*. Echocardiographic evaluation of cardiac resynchronization therapy: ready for routine clinical use? A critical appraisal. *J Am Coll Cardiol* 2004; 44: 1–9.

80 Bardy GH. Sudden Cardiac Death in Heart Failure Trial (SCD-HeFT). *American College of Cardiology 2004; Scientific Sessions: New Orleans*. 2004.

81 Kadish A, Dyer A, Daubert JP *et al*. Prophylactic defibrillator implantation in patients with nonischemic dilated cardiomyopathy. *N Engl J Med* 2004; 350: 2151–8.

82 Moss AJ, Hall WJ, Cannom DS *et al*. Improved survival with an implanted defibrillator in patients with coronary disease at high risk for ventricular arrhythmia. Multicenter Automatic Defibrillator Implantation Trial Investigators. *N Engl J Med* 1996; 335: 1933–40.

83 Walker S, Levy T, Paul VE. Dissection of the coronary sinus secondary to pacemaker lead manipulation. *Pacing Clin Electrophysiol* 2000; 23: 541–3.

84 Taieb J, Benchaa T, Foltzer E *et al*. Atrioventricular cross-talk in biventricular pacing: a potential cause of ventricular standstill. *Pacing Clin Electrophysiol* 2002; 25: 929–35.

85 Higgins SL, Yong P, Sheck D *et al*. Biventricular pacing diminishes the need for implantable cardioverter defibrillator therapy. Ventak CHF Investigators. *J Am Coll Cardiol* 2000; 36: 824–7.

86 Walker S, Levy TM, Rex S *et al*. Usefulness of suppression of ventricular arrhythmia by biventricular pacing in severe congestive cardiac failure. *Am J Cardiol* 2000; 86: 231–3.

87 Kies P, Bax JJ, Molhoek SG *et al*. Effect of left ventricular remodeling after cardiac resynchronization therapy on frequency of ventricular arrhythmias. *Am J Cardiol* 2004; 94: 130–2.

88 Guerra JM, Wu J, Miller JM, Groh WJ. Increase in ventricular tachycardia frequency after biventricular implantable cardioverter defibrillator upgrade. *J Cardiovasc Electrophysiol* 2003; 14: 1245–7.

89 Singh SN, Carson PE, Fisher SG. Nonsustained ventricular tachycardia in severe heart failure. *Circulation* 1997; 96: 3794–5.

90 Teerlink JR, Jalaluddin M, Anderson S *et al.* Ambulatory ventricular arrhythmias in patients with heart failure do not specifically predict an increased risk of sudden death. PROMISE (Prospective Randomized Milrinone Survival Evaluation) Investigators. *Circulation* 2000; 101: 40–6.

91 Al Ahmad A, Wang PJ, Homoud MK *et al.* Frequent ICD shocks due to double sensing in patients with bi-ventricular implantable cardioverter defibrillators. *J Interv Card Electrophysiol* 2003; 9: 377–81.

92 Liu BC, Villareal RP, Hariharan R *et al.* Inappropriate shock delivery and biventricular pacing cardiac defibrillators. *Tex Heart Inst J* 2003; 30: 45–9.

93 Tyers GF, Clark J, Wang Y *et al.* Coronary sinus lead extraction. *Pacing Clin Electrophysiol* 2003; 26: 524–6.

94 Nelson GS, Berger RD, Fetics BJ *et al.* Left ventricular or biventricular pacing improves cardiac function at diminished energy cost in patients with dilated cardiomyopathy and left bundle-branch block. *Circulation* 2000; 102: 3053–9.

95 Kim WY, Sogaard P, Mortensen PT *et al.* Three dimensional echocardiography documents haemodynamic improvement by biventricular pacing in patients with severe heart failure. *Heart* 2001; 85: 514–20.

96 Breithardt OA, Stellbrink C, Franke A *et al.* Acute effects of cardiac resynchronization therapy on left ventricular Doppler indices in patients with congestive heart failure. *Am Heart J* 2002; 143: 34–44.

97 Etienne Y, Mansourati J, Touiza A *et al.* Evaluation of left ventricular function and mitral regurgitation during left ventricular-based pacing in patients with heart failure. *Eur J Heart Fail* 2001; 3: 441–7.

98 Breithardt OA, Sinha AM, Schwammenthal E *et al.* Acute effects of cardiac resynchronization therapy on functional mitral regurgitation in advanced systolic heart failure. *J Am Coll Cardiol* 2003; 41: 765–70.

99 Ritter, P., Dib J-C, Lellevre T *et al.* Quick determination of the optimal AV delay at rest in patients paced in DDD mode for complete AV block (abstract). *JCPE* 1994; 163.

100 Perego GB, Chianca R, Facchini M *et al.* Simultaneous vs. sequential biventricular pacing in dilated cardiomyopathy: an acute hemodynamic study. *Eur J Heart Fail* 2003; 5: 305–13.

101 Sogaard P, Egeblad H, Pedersen AK *et al.* Sequential versus simultaneous biventricular resynchronization for severe heart failure: evaluation by tissue Doppler imaging. *Circulation* 2002; 106: 2078–84.

102 Oguz E, Dagdeviren B, Bilsel T *et al.* Echocardiographic prediction of long-term response to biventricular pacemaker in severe heart failure. *Eur J Heart Fail* 2002; 4: 83–90.

103 Blanc JJ, Bertault-Valls V, Fatemi M *et al.* Midterm benefits of left univentricular pacing in patients with congestive heart failure. *Circulation* 2004; 109: 1741–4.

CHAPTER 8

Pacing in special cases: hypertrophic cardiomyopathy, congenital heart disease

Martin Lowe, Mark Turner and Fiona Walker

Hypertrophic cardiomyopathy

Introduction

Hypertrophic cardiomyopathy, found in one in 500 of the general population, is the most common genetically transmitted cardiac disease. Current therapy is mainly directed at reducing in dynamic left ventricular (LV) outflow obstruction, improvement in diastolic relaxation, and prophylaxis against sudden cardiac death. Pacemaker implantation should be considered in those with conventional indications for pacing, that is, patients with postsurgical myomectomy and nonsurgical septal ablation with atrioventricular (AV) block, and those with outflow tract obstruction resistant to medical treatment.

Conventional indications for pacing

Hypertrophic cardiomyopathy may be complicated by sinus node disease and AV block, particularly in older patients. Complete AV block may also be seen in association with familial hypertrophic cardiomyopathy. In both groups of patients, pacemaker implantation is warranted according to conventional criteria (see the section on "Pacing/device therapy in the adult with congenital heart disease"). Chronotropic incompetence may be particularly troublesome in patients with sinus node disease, and exacerbated by pharmacological therapy such as β blockers and calcium antagonists. In these patients, implantation of a rate responsive pacemaker is likely to improve symptoms significantly.

Postsurgical myomectomy and nonsurgical septal ablation

Surgical myomectomy, performed for severely symptomatic patients with large outflow tract gradients (>50 mm Hg), may be complicated by postoperative AV block.[1] Conduction abnormalities are not uncommon, reflecting the site of muscle debaulking in the basal septum, with complete heart block requiring pacemaker implantation in around 5% of patients. In high volume centers with extensive surgical experience, implantation rates as low as 2% are achieved. Catheter-based septal ablation using alcohol, a newer technique, reduces outflow tract obstruction by producing a controlled myocardial infarct in the septal region. Complete heart block postablation was seen in 30–40% of patients in early series, but the use of myocardial contrast echocardiography to direct alcohol ablation has reduced the need for permanent pacing to less than 20% of patients.[2,3]

Reduction in outflow tract obstruction

The use of dual chamber pacing in patients with outflow tract obstruction alone remains controversial. While pacing can improve symptoms of outflow tract obstruction in some patients, outflow tract gradients are not consistently reduced, and objective measurements of exercise tolerance and myocardial workload often remain unchanged.

The potential beneficial mechanisms of dual chamber pacing in this setting include:

1 Reduction in systolic obstruction of the subaortic septum in the left ventricular outflow tract (LVOT) secondary to preexcitation of the right ventricular apex, producing a change in septal contraction. A reduction in LVOT obstruction from a reduced Venturi effect on the systolic anterior motion of the anterior mitral valve leaflet may also occur.

2 Reduction in systolic hypercontractility, secondary to a change in ventricular activation sequence, leading to a rightward shift of the LV end-systolic pressure–volume relationship with a reduction in myocardial work.

3 Reduction in functional mitral regurgitation secondary to reduced systolic anterior motion of the anterior mitral valve leaflet.

4 Improvement in diastolic function

5 Chronic remodeling of the left ventricle with regression of hypertrophy.

Early prospective studies in adults showed short-term improvement in symptoms, with a reduction in angina, dyspnea, palpitations, presyncope, and syncope in those undergoing dual chamber pacemaker implantation.[4,5] In these patients, an increase in exercise duration and decrease in New York Heart Association (NYHA) functional class were seen. This appeared to correlate with a reduction in LVOT gradient of around 50% and a corresponding increase in cardiac output and systemic pressures. Medium-term follow-up showed symptom elimination in one-third of patients, and significant improvement in one-half, with progressive reduction in LVOT gradient and continued improvement in NYHA score.[6] Formal quality of life assessment scores were also shown to improve by up to 40% with pacing. Intriguingly, in some patients there appeared to be a reversal in LV wall thickness with time, suggesting a remodeling process. Similar studies in the pediatric population also suggested that dual chamber pacemaker implantation may be useful in those with outflow tract obstruction, with a reduction in symptoms seen following pacing. This correlated with a reduction in LVOT gradient and pulmonary capillary wedge pressure.

However, blinded randomized crossover trials have shown more modest reductions in LVOT gradient reduction (20–30 mm Hg), with up to 40% of patients showing no change in gradient or exercise tolerance with DDD pacing.[7–10] In these studies, although symptoms of chest pain and dyspnea improved in most, a significant placebo response was seen with symptomatic relief in patients who were not actively paced. Some patients, however, experienced a worsening of symptoms during dual chamber pacing, and acute echocardiographic and hemodynamic assessment of systolic and diastolic function showed a significant decrease in cardiac output during dual chamber pacing at the shortest AV delay of 60 ms. Even while pacing at an optimal AV delay (longest AV delay associated with preexcitation of the ventricle), there was a similar trend with deterioration in both systolic and diastolic ventricular function. Medium-term studies also showed no evidence of ventricular remodeling following pacing.

Dual chamber pacing may benefit patients with midcavity obstruction, but this also remains controversial. Here obstruction at the level of papillary muscles may be associated with distal LV aneurysm formation and an adverse prognosis. The level of obstruction makes standard cardiac surgery more problematic, and patients often remain highly symptomatic despite medical treatment. For selected patients, dual chamber pacing may improve symptoms and reduce NYHA functional class.

Current American College of Cardiology/American Heart Association/North American Society of Pacing and Electrophysiology guidelines reflect the conflicting data regarding the benefit of dual chamber pacing in patients with obstructive hypertrophic cardiomyopathy.[11] This mode of therapy has been classified with a IIb indication for treatment, and it is thought that only around 10% of all patients are likely to be candidates. Those most likely to respond have one or more of the following conditions:
- Highly symptomatic despite conventional medication
- LVOT gradient > 50 mm Hg
- Significant functional mitral regurgitation
- Bradycardic indications for pacing
- High-risk surgical candidates, or unsuitable for alcohol septal ablation.

Patients who are not suitable for DDD pacing have:
- Concentric or apical hypertrophy, without outflow tract obstruction
- Structural mitral valve disease with significant regurgitation
- Fixed subvalvular aortic obstruction
- Uncontrolled atrial arrhythmias.

Following pacemaker implantation, the paced AV interval should be optimized, as there is substantial variation between patients in the interval required to maximize pacing via the right ventricular (RV) lead. Ventricular pacing should occur at all heart rates, bypassing intrinsic conduction via the AV node, which may require complex pacemaker programming. However, short AV delays may be associated with atrial contraction against a closed AV valve and reduction in cardiac output from loss of effective atrial transport. In patients with rapid intrinsic AV conduction, AV nodal blocking drugs may be required to slow conduction sufficiently to obtain preexcitation of the RV apex via the pacemaker. AV node ablation is occasionally required in resistant patients in sinus rhythm with rapid AV conduction or those with atrial fibrillation (AF) and uncontrolled ventricular rates. DDD pacing should be programmed appropriately with the assistance of Doppler dynamic measurements at different AV interval settings using echocardiography. Although invasive studies allow precise measurements of the optimal AV delay in individuals, and identify those patients with adverse hemodynamics acutely, they are usually not required in addition to noninvasive assessment.

Post-AV node ablation

Atrial fibrillation may affect up to 25% of patients with hypertrophic cardiomyopathy. Rapid ventricular rates during AF can lead to significant impairment of diastolic relaxation and symptoms and signs of heart failure. Adequate heart rate control may be suboptimal using pharmacological agents, and catheter ablation of focal AF triggers or AF substrate modification may not be successful. Under these circumstances AV nodal ablation followed by insertion of a rate-responsive ventricular pacemaker (in those with chronic AF) or dual chamber pacemaker (in those with paroxysmal AF) provides absolute control of ventricular rate, and improvement in cardiac function.

Biventricular pacing

Conventional indications for combined RV and LV pacing center on those patients with LV systolic dysfunction and evidence of conduction disease with a wide QRS complex. Preliminary evidence in patients with hypertrophic cardiomyopathy suggests that in some patients biventricular pacing (BVP) may reduce LVOT obstruction, but larger studies are required to confirm this. In those without obstruction, but who have a significant "restrictive" physiology with severely impaired diastolic function, BVP may improve cardiac output through beneficial effects on diastolic ventricular interaction (Figures 8.1 and 8.2). BVP may also improve systolic function in those patients with long standing hypertrophic cardiomyopathy who have marked LV dilatation and intraventricular or interventricular dyssynchrony.

Pacing/device therapy in the adult with congenital heart disease

Introduction

In the current era ~90% of those born with congenital heart disease (CHD) survive to adulthood. There will soon be more adults than children with CHD and for several conditions life expectancy is approaching that of the normal population. Of the estimated 20 000 adults with CHD in the United Kingdom, around 2–4% of them will require pacemaker implantation and for most the

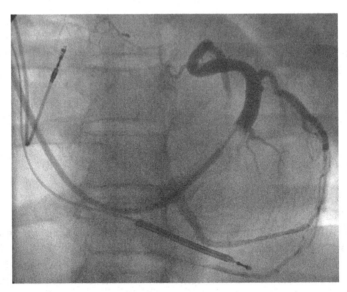

Figure 8.1 Coronary sinus angiography in a patient with hypertrophic cardiomyopathy. A suitable anterolateral branch is identified for LV pacing.

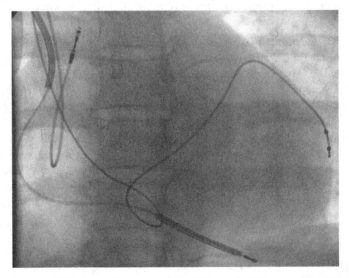

Figure 8.2 LV lead placement in an anterolateral branch of the coronary sinus.

first implant is in adulthood, with only ~30% of implantations occurring in childhood.[12]

The indications for pacemaker/device intervention continue to expand, but at present it is divided almost equally between perioperative AV block (at the time of initial operation or re-do surgery) and the development of late sinus node or AV nodal disease often years after surgery. Repaired atrial septal defects (ASDs), ventricular septal defects (VSDs), and atrioventricular septal defects (AVSDs) comprise around 30% of this paced population. Patients with a Mustard or Senning repair for transposition of the great arteries (TGA) and those with congenitally corrected transposition (CCTGA) account for ~20%, repaired tetralogy of Fallot (TOF) account for ~15%, and a substantial proportion (~17%) have complex anatomic CHD, including single ventricle anatomy and Fontan palliations.[12]

The onset of atrial and ventricular tachyarrhythmias deserves special consideration in this patient population, as it may herald hemodynamic problems. All patients with new arrhythmias should therefore always be investigated with transthoracic echo (TTE) or transesophageal echo (TOE), cardiac catheterization, and exercise testing. If hemodynamic problems are identified these should be treated prior to electrophysiological assessment or device therapy.

Special considerations in the grown up congenital heart (GUCH) disease population

Duration of pacing

Adults with CHD who require pacemaker or implantable defibrillator therapy have a lifelong need for reintervention and follow-up. Given the possibility that right ventricular (RV) apical pacing may be detrimental to ventricular function, alternative strategies must be considered including pacing the RV septum or using BVP.

Venous access

While the transvenous approach for lead implantation is preferred, this is not always technically feasible because of natural anatomic variation, including venous abnormalities; for example, persistent left superior vena cava (SVC), left atrial (LA) isomerism, as well as reparative or palliative surgeries {e.g. Glenn shunts [SVC to pulmonary artery (PA)], Fontan [right atrium to PA] or Mustard repair}.

Left SVC. A left SVC characteristically drains into the posterior part of the coronary sinus in the AV groove. This makes lead manipulations difficult but not impossible. Alternatively, it may drain directly into the left atrium, causing a right-to-left shunt, which poses a thromboembolic risk.

LA isomerism. Both atria are morphologic left atria. There may be no sinus node [a right atrial (RA) structure] and atrial bradycardia. There may be no continuity between the IVC and the atrium, and blood may drain via an Azygos continuation into the SVC.[13] This may pose problems if temporary pacing is attempted from the femoral vein.

Fontan operation. An RA–PA/AP Fontan (Figure 8.3) allows access to the coronary sinus from the right atrium for ventricular pacing, however, in a lateral tunnel or extracardiac Fontan [total cavo-pulmonary connection (TCPC)]

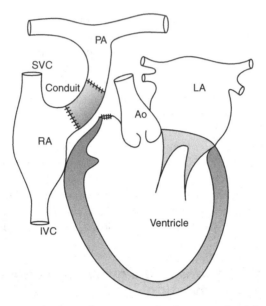

Figure 8.3 AP Fontan. There is a direct connection between the right atrium and pulmonary artery.

(Figure 8.4) the coronary sinus usually drains to the left artium and is therefore not accessible, unless a fenestration has been left by the surgeon.

Intracardiac shunts

Intracardiac shunts are associated with a risk of paradoxical embolism, a risk that may be increased in the presence of endocardial pacing leads. This risk has not been quantified, but anticoagulation or antiplatelet therapy should be considered. Oxygen saturations or bubble contrast echocardiography (TTE) should be performed prior to implantation to look for any intracardiac shunting.

Shunts may also make lead implantation more challenging. Leads may pass inadvertently through septal defects to systemic chambers. Lead position should be checked in oblique X-ray views and paced QRS morphology should be checked ideally in lead V_1.

Septal defects/intracardiac shunts are present in the following: Ebstein's anomaly (shunt at atrial level), atrial isomerism, fenestrated Fontan, Mustard repair with a baffle leak, patent foramen ovale/ASD/ VSD.

Lead selection

The morphology of the target chamber determines lead choice. Active-fixation leads are often required in dilated chambers and when the smooth-walled sub-pulmonary morphologic left ventricle is paced. Catheter-based lead delivery systems offer additional flexibility for implanting leads in these complex hearts.

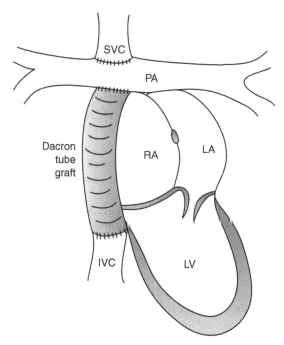

Figure 8.4 Extracardiac Fontan or TCPC. Systemic venous blood drains directly to the pulmonary arteries, bypassing the right heart.

Epicardial pacing

For some patients with difficult venous access or thromboembolic risk associated with endocardial pacing leads, epicardial leads may be necessary. Epicardial pacing in these patients is not without some risk/complications and it must be remembered that these patients have had multiple previous sternotomies. Modern steroid eluting epicardial leads however do provide an acceptable alternative to endocardial pacing.[14] Thoracoscopic lead delivery has been used as an alternative mode of lead placement with success.

Specific congenital heart lesions commonly associated with pacemaker/device therapy

Repaired isolated ventricular septal defect (VSD)

Common indications for pacing. Perioperative AV block. More common following repair of perimembranous defects.

Venous access. Venous access is normal; access for pacing is usually straightforward with no special considerations.

Repaired AVSD

Common indications for pacing. Perioperative AV block and late atrial arrhythmias.

Venous access. Usually straightforward but residual intracardiac shunts may be present.

Atrioventricular septal defects encompass a spectrum of lesions caused by abnormal endocardial cushion development. Adults are likely to have had surgery in childhood and require follow-up for surveillance of residua and sequelae relating to this surgery (left AV valve regurgitation, subaortic stenosis, and late atrial arrhythmias).

Mustard/Senning operations for transposition of great vessels

Prior to the arterial switch operation (1976), patients born with TGA underwent surgical venous redirection of blood flow at atrial level, to physiologically correct blood flow (Mustard or Senning operations). In the Mustard operation, pathways or "baffles" made of Dacron or pericardium, divert blood flow (Figure 8.5), whereas in the Senning operation, infoldings of the atrial walls themselves are used. Both operations lead to extensive atrial scarring.

Common indications for pacing. Perioperative AV block, late AV block, late sinus node dysfunction (sinus bradycardia, sinus pauses, and intermittent nodal

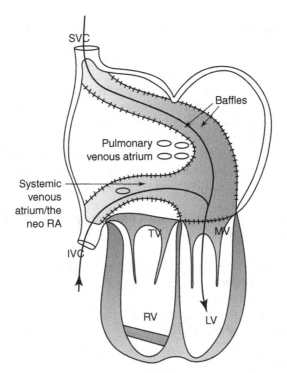

Figure 8.5 Mustard Repair for TGA. Baffles direct the venous return to the opposite ventricle – a "venous switch."

rhythm) and atrial tachyarrhythmias. Pacing is indicated if there is high-grade AV block or if there is sinus node dysfunction and symptoms of effort intolerance or presyncope, in the presence of chronotropic incompetence. Some may require backup pacing to facilitate adequate medical treatment of atrial tachyarrhythmias. Pacemakers with atrial antitachycardia functions are being more widely employed.

Venous access. Standard venous access, with the proviso that SVC pathway obstruction has been excluded. If there is any narrowing of the SVC baffle it should be stented prior to (or at the time of) pacemaker implantation. Active fixation leads should be used. The A-lead is positioned in the roof of the neo-right atrium (morphologic left atrium) and the V-lead is positioned in the subpulmonary ventricle (morphologic left ventricle) having traversed the venous baffles and mitral valve (Figures 8.6 and 8.7).

Repaired tetralogy of Fallot

Patients with repaired TOF have undergone closure of a VSD and resection of RV outflow tract obstruction, which may have required a transannular patch. The important residua and sequelae of this operation are pulmonary

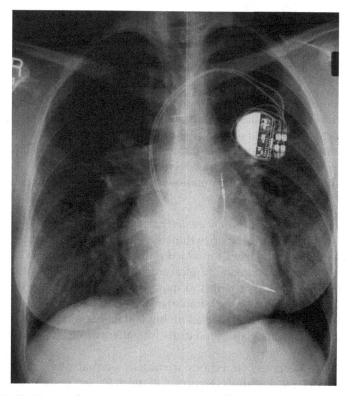

Figure 8.6 PA X-rays of a Mustard patient with a dual chamber pacing system.

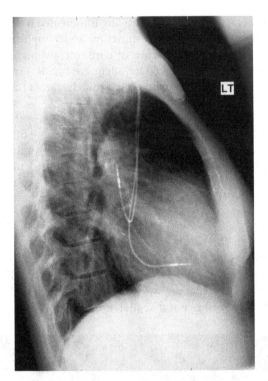

Figure 8.7 Lateral X-ray of the same Mustard patient showing the posterior position of the leads.

regurgitation (PR), late ventricular arrhythmias, and sudden death. AV block may contribute to the sudden death risk as prolonged perioperative AV block is a risk factor for sudden death.[15] Significant PR causes RV dilatation, which is a substrate for ventricular arrhythmias and sudden death. Sudden death is, however, rare and risk stratification is based on many factors.[16] Re-do surgery and pulmonary homograft implantation may also be necessary over long-term follow-up.

Common indications for pacing/implantable cardioverter-defibrillator. Perioperative AV block and late ventricular arrhythmias. Patients with high-grade perioperative AV block require pacing. Sustained ventricular tachycardia (VT) may also be seen. RV dilatation, stretch, surgical scarring, and slow ventricular activation contribute to reentry circuits. VT may be poorly tolerated due to impaired RV function and PR. Those with important PR should have pulmonary valve implantation and surgical cryoablation. Implantable cardioverter-defibrillator (ICD) implantation may also protect at-risk patients from further VT and or sudden death.

Venous access. Venous connections are usually normal. Many patients have severe RA and RV dilatation (Figures 8.8 and 8.9) and myocardial scarring makes lead implantation technically challenging.

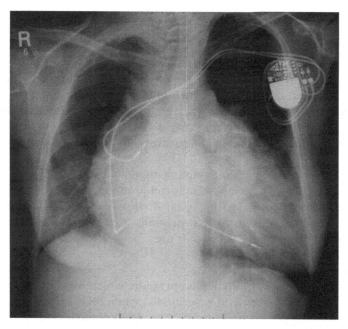

Figure 8.8 PA X-ray of a patient with severe pulmonary regurgitation and right heart failure following TOF repair.

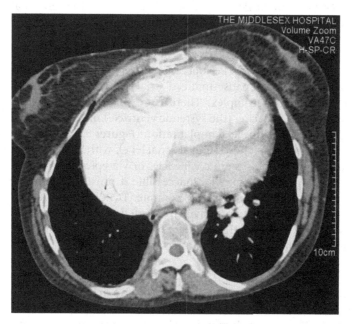

Figure 8.9 CT scan of the same patient as Figure 8.8 demonstrating massive dilatation of the right atrium and ventricle making atrial lead positioning more challenging.

Congenital complete heart block

Congenital complete heart block (CCHB) is rare and is associated with maternal anti-Ro or anti-La antinuclear antibodies that damage the conducting system.[17] Patients may develop heart failure due to a myopathic process associated with CCHB or alternatively long-term RV apical or epicardial pacing at high rates (that may cause dyssynchronous contraction and heart failure). BVP can reverse ventricular dilatation and heart failure. Use of an RV septal lead position rather than the apex may decrease the chance of heart failure; however, optimal lead position and pacing mode is yet to be clarified.[18]

Common indications for pacing. Symptomatic bradycardia (e.g. poor exercise capacity, presyncope, or hemodynamic compromise), ventricular dysfunction (ideally avoiding RV apical pacing or rapid rates), and low cardiac output.[19]

Venous access. These are usually structurally normal hearts and therefore a conventional transvenous approach is used.

Fontan patients

There are three main versions of this operation, which was designed to bypass the subpulmonary ventricle. It is performed when biventricular repair is not possible; for example, tricuspid atresia. The atriopulmonary (AP) Fontan uses a direct connection of the RA appendage to the PA (Figure 8.3). A lateral tunnel Fontan uses a Glenn anastomosis (SVC to RPA) with a passage from RA to direct IVC blood to the PA. The extracardiac TCPC uses a Glenn anastomosis, in combination with an extracardiac conduit (usually Dacron) to connect the IVC and PA (Figure 8.4).

Common indications for pacing. Perioperative sinus node dysfunction, late sinus node dysfunction,[20] and pause-induced atrial tachyarrhythmias.

Venous access. Highly complex. There is no subpulmonary right ventricle, therefore access to V-pacing (the systemic ventricle) may be achieved in some patients by coronary sinus lead implantation (Figures 8.10 and 8.11), via passage of a lead through a fenestration at atrial level, with lead implantation into the endocardium of the systemic ventricle, or via epicardial lead placement. Even atrial endocardium may be inaccessible if prosthetic tubes have been used for surgical reconstruction; for example, TCPC Fontan. It is also worth appreciating that these patients have an elevated venous pressure, with mean RA pressures of 10–14 mm Hg. Bleeding problems at the time of implantation should therefore be expected and anticipated.

Congenitally corrected transposition of the great arteries

This condition is also known as double discordance or ventricular inversion (Figure 8.12). The right atrium drains via a mitral valve into the left ventricle, which connects to PA and pulmonary venous blood returns to the left atriums via a tricuspid valve into the RV and then to the aorta. As the right ventricle is

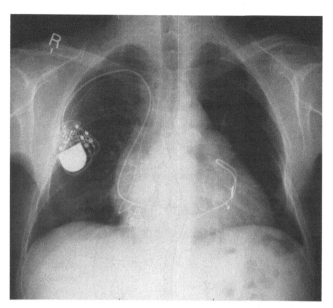

Figure 8.10 PA and lateral X-rays of a patient with an AP Fontan with sinus bradycardia and AV block. The ventricular lead was placed a long way into the coronary sinus in an anterior branch. A catheter-delivered lead screwed into the hugely enlarged right atrium adjacent to the RA-PA connection can also be seen.

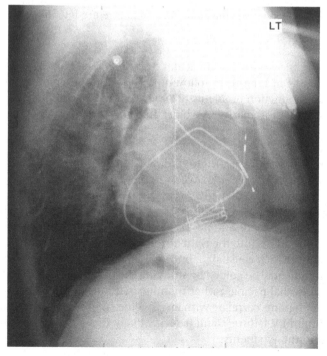

Figure 8.11 (See text for details.)

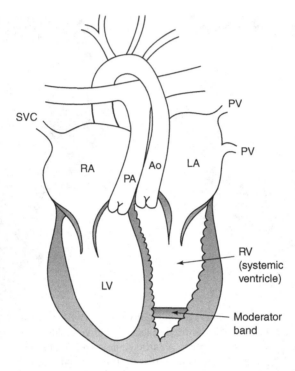

Figure 8.12 CCTGA. The ventricular malposition ensures that the systemic venous blood drains to the lungs and the pulmonary venous return is to the systemic (right) ventricle.

now the systemic ventricle, ventricular dysfunction and heart failure are seen over the course of long-term follow-up. There is a progressive tendency to develop AV conduction problems (2% per year risk of complete heart block). The first presentation may be AV block in some patients.

Common indication for pacing. High-grade AV block.

Venous access and lead positions. Access to the right atrium is normal (although the right atrium may be dilated). Access to the subpulmonary ventricle (morphological left ventricle) is via the mitral valve. This is usually straightforward but active fixation leads should be used. BVP is technically feasible as the coronary sinus drains into the right atrium. The anatomy of the distal branching pattern of the CS is usually abnormal and venography is mandatory. CS lead positioning may be guided by studying the timing of lead tip electrograms during endocardial pacing, rather than by anatomic position. The lateness of lead tip electrograms correlate with improvements in synchrony during resynchronization in LV failure[21] and it seems likely that similar mechanisms will be present in these patients.

Conclusion

Pacing/device implantation in this unique and heterogenous patient population is best performed by cardiologists with an understanding of the anatomy and physiology of congenital heart lesions. The indications for pacing, implant techniques, and postimplant pacemaker management differ from patients with structurally normal hearts. A detailed knowledge of the structural abnormalities and any prior surgeries are essential not only when considering the indications for pacing, but also in choosing the necessary equipment and techniques that need to be employed to achieve optimal pacing. The long-term implications of pacing/device therapy with the attendant need for reintervention and follow-up, potentially over a time course in excess of 60 years, are as yet unknown.

References

1 Merrill WH, Friesinger GC, Graham TP *et al.* Long-lasting improvement after septal myectomy for hypertrophic obstructive cardiomyopathy. *Ann Thorac Surg* 2000; 69: 1732–5.

2 Nagueh SF, Ommen SR, Lakkis NM *et al.* Comparison of ethanol septal reduction therapy with surgical myectomy for the treatment of hypertrophic obstructive cardiomyopathy. *J Am Coll Cardiol* 2001; 38: 1701–6.

3 Chang SM, Nagueh SF, Spencer WH III *et al.* Complete heart block: determinants and clinical impact in patients with hypertrophic obstructive cardiomyopathy undergoing nonsurgical septal reduction therapy. *J Am Coll Cardiol* 2003; 42: 296–300.

4 Jeanrenaud X, Goy JJ, Kappenberger L. Effects of dual-chamber pacing in hypertrophic obstructive cardiomyopathy. *Lancet* 1992; 339: 1318–23.

5 Fananapazir L, Cannon RO, Tripodi D *et al.* Impact of dual-chamber permanent pacing in patients with obstructive hypertrophic cardiomyopathy with symptoms refractory to verapamil and beta-adrenergic blocker therapy. *Circulation* 1992; 85: 2149–61.

6 Fananapazir L, Epstein ND, Curiel RV *et al.* Long-term results of dual-chamber (DDD) pacing in obstructive hypertrophic cardiomyopathy. Evidence for progressive symptomatic and hemodynamic improvement and reduction of left ventricular hypertrophy. *Circulation* 1994; 90: 2731–42.

7 Nishimura RA, Hayes DL, Ilstrup DM *et al.* Effect of dual chamber pacing on systolic and diastolic function in patients with hypertrophic cardiomyopathy. Acute Doppler echocardiographic and catheterisation hemodynamic study. *J Am Coll Cardiol* 1996; 27: 421–30.

8 Nishimura RA, Trusty JM, Hayes DL *et al.* Dual chamber pacing for hypertrophic cardiomyopathy. A randomized, double blind, crossover trial. *J Am Coll Cardiol* 1997; 29: 435–41.

9 Kappenberger L, Linde C, Daubert C *et al.* Pacing in hypertrophic obstructive cardiomyopathy. A randomized crossover study. PIC Study Group. *Eur Heart J* 1997; 18: 1249–56.

10 Maron BJ, Nishimura RA, McKenna WJ *et al.* (For the M-PATHY Study Investigators). Assessment of permanent dual-chamber pacing as a treatment for

drug-refractory symptomatic patients with obstructive hypertrophic cardiomy-opathy. A randomised double blind, crossover study (M-PATHY). *Circulation* 1999; 99: 2927–33.

11 ACC/AHA/NASPE 2002 guideline update for implantation of cardiac pacemakers and antiarrhythmia devices. *Circulation* 2002; 106: 2145–61.

12 Walker F, Siu SC, Woods S *et al.* Long-term outcomes of cardiac pacing in adults with congenital heart disease. *J Am Coll Cardiol* 2004; 43: 1894–901.

13 Wu WH, Wang JK, Lin JL *et al.* Cardiac rhythm disturbances in patients with left atrial isomerism. *Pacing Clin Electrophysiol* 2001; 24: 1631–8.

14 Cohen MI, Bush DM, Vetter VL *et al.* Permanent epicardial pacing in pediatric patients: seventeen years experience and 1200 out-patient visits. *Circulation* 2001; 103: 2585–90.

15 Hokanson JS, Moller JH. Significance of early transient complete heart block as a predictor of sudden death late after operative repair of tetralogy of fallot. *Am J Cardiol* 2001; 87: 1271–7.

16 Steeds RP, Oakley D. Predicting late sudden death from ventricular arrhythmia in patients following surgical repair of tetralogy of Fallot. *QJM* 2004; 97: 7–13.

17 Hu K, Qu Y, Yue Y *et al.* Functional basis of sinus bradycardia in congenital heart block. *Circ Res* 2004; 94: e32–8.

18 Horenstein MS, Karpawich PP. Pacemaker syndrome in the young: do children need dual chamber as the initial pacing mode. *Pacing Clin Electrophysiol* 2004; 27: 600–5.

19 ACC/AHA/NASPE 2002 guideline update for implantation of cardiac pacemakers and antiarrhythmia devices: summary article. *Circulation* 2002; 106: 2145–61.

20 Dilawar M, Bradley SM, Saul JP *et al.* Sinus node dysfunction after intraatrial lateral tunnel and extracardiac conduit Fontan procedures. *Pediatr Cardiol* 2003; 24: 284–8.

21 Turner MS, Bleasdale RA, Vinereanu D *et al.* Electrical and mechanical components of dyssynchrony in heart failure patients with normal QRS duration and left bundle-branch block: impact of left and biventricular pacing. *Circulation* 2004; 109: 2544–9.

CHAPTER 9
Lead problems, device infections, and lead extraction

Richard Schilling and Simon Sporton

Introduction

Malfunction of a pacemaker or implantable cardioverter-defibrillator (ICD) pulse generator is fortunately rare. Device malfunction is almost invariably due to a problem with a lead, its connection with the pulse generator or its interface with the myocardium. It is important that everyone involved with device implantation and follow-up has a thorough understanding of lead problems in order that the incidence of such problems is minimized and that when they occur, they are recognized promptly and managed appropriately.

Device infection occurs in every implanting center and may be life threatening. Apparently minor wound infections are frequently mismanaged due to a lack of understanding of the potential danger of device infection and failure to refer early to a specialist device center. The causes, presentation, and management of device infection are considered in this chapter.

Finally, we discuss the indications for lead extraction and describe the developments that have rendered percutaneous lead extraction the technique of choice in almost every case.

Lead problems

Lead malfunction may result from problems with
- the lead connector
- the lead body
- the electrode–myocardium interface
- interactions between two or more adjacent leads.

Lead connector malfunction
The most common problem in lead connector malfunction is failure to tighten one of the set-screws in the device header at implant. This should be recognized easily by extremely high pacing or shock impedance associated with failure of sensing/pacing or defibrillation. The problem can be avoided by routinely checking lead parameters at implant, not only via the pacing system analyzer but also via the generator using a sterile telemetry wand.

Lead body malfunction

Problems with the lead body itself may occur as a result of damage to the insulation, the conductor coil(s), or to lead shaping mechanisms. Causes include:

1 Damage by instruments at the time of implantation or generator change: lead insulation materials are exquisitely sensitive to any trauma from surgical instruments. Damage to the lead insulation at implant may not cause overt insulation failure but may introduce a weakness that results in insulation failure several years later.

2 Anchoring sutures: although anchoring sutures should be tight enough to prevent lead migration at the point of vascular access, excessively tight sutures can result in damage to the lead. Failure to use the protective collar and suturing the lead directly also leads to a high incidence of insulation damage. Some device implanters do not use anchor sutures, particularly when implanting in the pediatric population but this may result in a higher incidence of lead displacement.

3 Lead crush and fracture between the clavicle and first rib (Figure 9.1): the risk of subclavian crush is minimized by the use of the cephalic vein or a more lateral puncture into the axillary vein as it crosses the lateral border of the first rib.

Lead disruption is more common with pediatric device implants. In some cases, this has been attributed to large traction forces on the lead as a result of tethering by fibrous tissue and growth of the thorax.

The hallmark of insulation failure is a sudden reduction in pacing impedance. In the case of *unipolar* leads escape of current at the site of insulation failure may result in local muscle twitch. Loss of myocardial capture may also occur due to short-circuiting. Failure of the internal insulation of a *bipolar* lead may allow the development of contact potentials between the inner and outer conductor coils resulting in oversensing and either inhibition of bradycardia pacing or inappropriate tachycardia therapies. Short-circuiting may result in loss of myocardial capture and sensing may be compromised.

Disruption of the lead conductor is characteristically associated with a sudden rise in pacing impedance with variable effects on pacing and sensing (Figure 9.2). Contact potentials may occur between the fractured ends of the conductor. There may be marked variations in lead parameters over short periods of time and with changes of body position.

It is important to note that when following up suspected lead insulation or conductor problems, changes in impedance or electrogram appearance are often intermittent and that it may be necessary to ask the patient to perform a variety of maneuvers to reveal the problem.

A specific problem affects the Telectronics Accufix and Encor leads. These are J-shaped bipolar active fixation atrial leads, of which more than 60 000 were implanted worldwide during the late 1980s and early 1990s. The Accufix lead incorporates a J-shaped retention wire between the outer insulation and

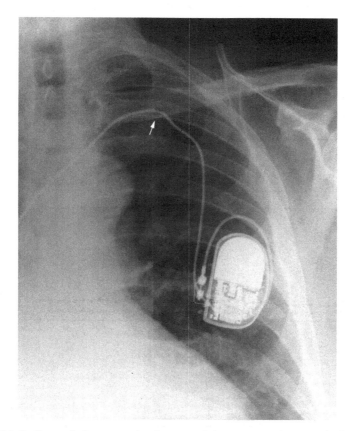

Figure 9.1 Radiograph demonstrating fracture of the outer conductor coil of a bipolar pacing lead between the clavicle and first rib (arrow).

the outer conductor coil, welded distally to the proximal ring electrode. The Encor lead also incorporates a J-shaped retention wire although in this lead the retention wire is contained within the inner conductor coil and welded to the tip electrode distally. The retention wires of both leads have a tendency to fracture and perforate the outer insulation where they may damage surrounding structures or embolize (Figure 9.3). The electrical parameters of Accufix leads are unaffected by retention wire fracture. The Accufix Research Institute was established in 1996 to collect data and provide clinicians with information and guidelines for the management of patients with Accufix and Encor leads. Management revolves around regular fluoroscopic surveillance and, for some patients, lead extraction. The details may be viewed at www.accufix.com. It is of note that more people have died worldwide as a result of extraction of Accufix leads than have died as a result of fracture of the retention wire, so extraction is not without its risks.

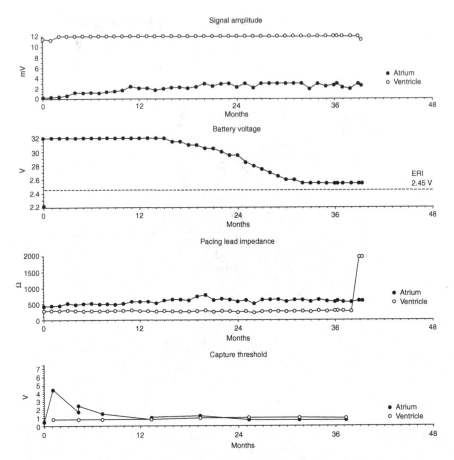

Figure 9.2 Time trend graphs from a dual chamber ICD showing a sudden marked impedance rise in the ventricular lead to over 2000 Ω as a result of conductor fracture, 3 years after device implantation. Sensed R-wave amplitude has fallen from >12 mV to 11.4 mV. Capture threshold has not been measured since the impedance rise.

Electrode–myocardium interface

Immediate problems seen within hours or a few days of implant include lead displacement, and myocardial penetration and perforation. Each of these complications is usually recognized by a marked deterioration of both the capture threshold and the amplitude of the sensed electrogram. There may or may not be any radiological evidence of lead displacement. Pericarditis and/or a pericardial effusion suggest that perforation has occurred. The treatment is lead repositioning. If penetration or perforation are suspected then the facilities to detect and drain a pericardial effusion should be immediately available.

An acute inflammatory response occurs at the electrode myocardial interface with both active fixation and tined leads. The inflammatory response

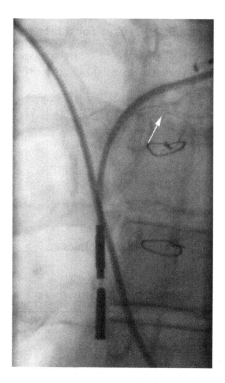

Figure 9.3 Radiograph demonstrating fracture of the J-shaped retention wire of a Telectronics Accufix atrial lead (arrow). The retention wire has perforated the outer insulation.

organizes gradually, encapsulating the lead tip in fibrous tissue that binds the lead but separates the lead tip from the endocardium. The extent of the inflammatory response may be reduced considerably by the use of steroid-eluting leads. As a result of the inflammatory reaction, the capture threshold typically rises following lead implant, reaching a peak during the first six weeks before falling back to a chronic capture threshold that is usually a little higher than that seen at implant. The changes in capture threshold during the first few weeks are typically mirrored by a reduction in the amplitude of the sensed electrogram and a reduction in pacing impedance. These early changes of pacing parameters are attenuated by the use of steroid-eluting leads. An exaggerated foreign body response at the electrode–myocardial interface may account for a late rise in the capture threshold.

A variety of other causes exist for a late rise in capture threshold (Box 9.1).

Interaction between leads

Contact potentials are generated when electrodes from adjacent leads touch each other, between the inner and outer conductors of a bipolar lead where there is inner insulation failure or between the ends of a fractured conductor. Where the decision is made to implant a new lead in the same chamber as an existing lead, the risk of contact potentials can be minimized by the use of active fixation leads with the electrodes positioned away from the

Box 9.1 Causes for a late rise in capture threshold

New or progressive heart disease
  Acute myocardial ischemia
  Infarction
  Cardiomyopathy
Metabolic
  Hypoxia
  Hypercarbia
  Metabolic acidosis
  Metabolic alkalosis
  Hyperkalemia
  Hyperglycemia
Drugs
  Class I antiarrhythmics
  Sotalol
  Amiodarone
Defibrillation and diathermy

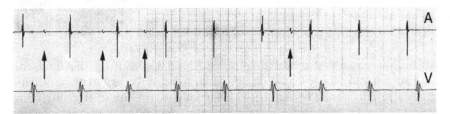

Figure 9.4 Atrial (A) and ventricular (V) electrograms recorded from a dual chamber defibrillator. The brief potentials unrelated to the cardiac cycle seen on the atrial channel (arrows) are contact potentials between the ring electrode of the atrial lead and proximal shock coil of a dual coil defibrillation lead.

existing electrodes. Lead tip position should be confirmed in more than one fluoroscopic plane. Furthermore, the use of defibrillation leads with an integrated bipole should be avoided in this situation. The right ventricular shock coil forms the anode of the pace-sense bipole of these leads, providing a large surface area for contact with other electrodes in the same chamber. Contact potentials have a characteristic appearance: brief, often multiple potentials usually unrelated to the cardiac cycle and often intermittent (Figure 9.4). These potentials may be sensed as cardiac events leading to inappropriate bradycardia or tachycardia therapy. It is sometimes possible to manage the problem of contact potentials without reintervention. Where the problem is contact with the proximal ring electrode of a bipolar lead, programming to unipolar sensing, so that the proximal electrode is not used, may solve the

problem. In the case of bipolar leads with internal insulation failure, reprogramming a ventricular lead to the unipolar sensing will also overcome the
problem. However, the integrity of the lead is compromised and for most
patients lead replacement is indicated, with or without extraction of the
failed lead.

Device infection

Although device infection by hematogenous spread from a remote source
is well documented, most infections occur as a result of wound contamination at the time of implantation or erosion through the skin, typically
with *Staphylococcus aureus* and *Staphylococcus epidermidis*. Poor surgical technique predisposes to infection from long procedure times, inadequate aseptic
technique, and hematoma formation providing a culture medium. Furthermore, inadequate pocket formation and wound closure may lead to pressure
necrosis of the overlying skin and subcutaneous tissue resulting in device
erosion.

Infection of an implanted device may present in a variety of ways:

1 Erosion of device material typically occurs with no local or systemic signs
of infection although bacterial colonization is inevitable.

2 Acute pocket infections may present with a purulent effusion, cellulitis, or
both.

3 Occasionally, a chronic draining sinus develops with little or no evidence
of inflammation unless drainage is prevented.

4 Septicemia and endocarditis may occur with no signs whatsoever of pocket
infection. A high index of suspicion is necessary in patients with implanted
devices or either of these conditions, especially when *Staphylococci* are
isolated or there has been a recent device-related procedure.

Although antibiotic therapy may lead to short-term resolution of clinical
infection and improvement of laboratory tests of infection, it will not erad-
icate the organisms completely and recurrence is inevitable. Consequently,
there is no place for antibiotic therapy alone. In cases of erosion and infection apparently localized to the pocket, a strategy of antibiotic therapy and
conservative surgery involving debridement of infected tissue, topical anti-
septic agents, antibiotics, and preservation of the device has been evaluated.[1]
Unfortunately, the recurrence rate with this strategy is high (over 50%)
and such an approach is unjustified. Delaying definitive treatment may
allow life-threatening septicemia to occur or, in the case of an early postimplant infection, turn an easy lead extraction into a difficult one because
it will allow fibrosis to develop around the leads. The development of lead
extraction techniques that are associated with high success rates and low complication rates has led to the recommendation that device infection should
be managed by aggressive antibiotic therapy and complete removal of the
device, all foreign bodies, and infected tissue. All confirmed and strongly
suspected device infections should be referred to a specialist pacing center for full evaluation and assessment. Bacteriological samples should be

taken before instituting antibiotic therapy and clinicians are strongly advised not to undertake diagnostic aspiration of collections as this may introduce new organisms into a sterile pocket or further contaminate an existing infection.

The patient presenting with a device infection should be admitted to hospital immediately. Intravenous antibiotic therapy should commence as soon as blood and wound swabs have been taken for culture. The antibiotics should be broad spectrum but should provide good cover for *Staphylococci*, and early consultation with a microbiologist is advisable. Evidence of endocarditis should be sought as this will govern the duration of antibiotic therapy. If septicemia is confirmed or strongly suspected, device extraction should be performed without delay. In other circumstances, device extraction may be deferred until local and systemic signs of infection have resolved with antibiotic therapy because there is a low incidence of septicemic shock associated with manipulating infected pacing systems. In addition to removal of all device components (see below) and sutures, inflammatory and necrotic tissue should be debrided. Primary closure of the wound is usually satisfactory and should be obtained using interrupted nonabsorbable sutures through the skin and subcutaneous tissue; the rationale being that following suture removal no foreign body remains in the wound. A closed drainage system in the wound may be used for a short period to prevent fluid collection. Wherever possible the use of temporary pacing wires should be avoided as infection may be perpetuated in this fashion. If a temporary pacing wire is necessary the internal jugular vein on the side of device explantation should be used wherever possible to avoid contaminating the opposite side, which will be used for implantation of a new device. Following device extraction, the route and duration of antibiotic therapy is determined by the patient's clinical progress. It is sensible to observe the patient clinically and with laboratory indices of inflammation for several days off antibiotics before implanting a new device.

Device extraction

Introduction

Following implantation, pacemaker or defibrillator generators and leads become surrounded by fibrous tissue, which in the case of the leads will bind them to the heart and great veins. The degree of tethering varies widely and although there is a correlation between the duration of implant and the ease of removal, it is safest to assume that any lead implanted for more than 3 months may be firmly tethered. The speed and degree of tethering is often greater in younger patients. An attempt at lead extraction by tugging the lead should be avoided as it may cause disruption of the lead preventing safe percutaneous lead extraction, avulsion of the myocardium, or irreversible inversion of the right ventricle or atrium (it is easier to pull a lead through a fibrous sleeve than push it back again when it does not come out!).

Lead construction

An understanding of lead construction is important. Unipolar pacemaker leads consist of a single helical conductor coil linking the lead connector to the tip electrode. The coil has a central lumen and is surrounded by a layer of silicone rubber or polyurethane insulation. Bipolar pacing leads have an additional coaxial outer coil connected to the proximal ring electrode. There are layers of insulation between the inner and outer coils and surrounding the outer coil. The construction of defibrillator leads is more complex and there is variation between manufacturers. However, all defibrillator leads have a tip electrode for pacing and sensing. For every type of lead, it is the coil leading to the tip electrode that must be identified and exposed during lead extraction by the superior approach.

Planning the procedure

Accurate knowledge of the hardware to be extracted is invaluable and is usually possible from a combination of pacing clinic records, the patient's device identification card, a chest X-ray, and readily available reference manuals listing leads from every manufacturer and relating model number to a description of the lead. The important information is:
- How many leads are there
- How long have they been implanted
- Are they unipolar or bipolar
- Do they have tined or active fixation
- Were they implanted via the cephalic or subclavian vein.

It is also important to consider the indication for device implantation and to assess the patient's underlying rhythm. Where the indication for removal is infection, echocardiography should be used to look for vegetations on the leads as these may be considered an indication for surgical lead removal.[2] Lead extraction may occasionally tear a great vein or the heart wall and facilities for emergency pericardiocentesis and immediate access to cardiothoracic surgery are mandatory. Blood should be grouped before the procedure although routine crossmatching seems unjustified. The procedure can be extremely painful: intravenous moderate sedation with a combination of benzodiazepines and opiates is a reasonable alternative to general anesthesia where there is experience in its safe administration. There is a strong case for continuous arterial pressure monitoring in order to rapidly detect major intrathoracic bleeding or cardiac tamponade. A 7 or 8 French femoral venous sheath allows the placement of a temporary pacing wire as well as the administration of drugs and large volumes of fluid if necessary. Continuous electrocardiogram ECG monitoring and immediate access to a defibrillator are mandatory.

Lead mobilization

It is essential that each lead to be explanted is freed of all binding material in the form of fibrous tissue, lead collars, and sutures proximal to the vein entry site. The lead connector often prevents the lead being pulled through a sheath of fibrous tissue. In this situation the lead connector of tined leads may be cut off. In the case of active fixation leads, the lead should be mobilized fully and the active fixation mechanism retracted before the lead is cut.

Extraction from the superior or inferior approach?

Once the generator has been removed and the leads freed, a decision can be made about the approach to lead extraction.[3] This largely depends on operator experience but factors that may influence the decision include the degree of fibrous lead adhesions: pulling the lead through from below may be easier than extensive subclavian dissection. Conversely, the superior approach may be preferred when dealing with large leads, such as defibrillator leads, because the lead has to be withdrawn and doubled up into a femoral lead extraction sheath.

Superior approach lead extraction

Exposing the inner coil

The first step is to expose the inner coil in order to introduce a locking stylet. The lead is then cut with lead clippers.

Locking stylets

A locking stylet is advanced to the tip of the inner conductor coil whereupon a locking mechanism is activated that fixes the stylet to the conductor coil, allowing traction to be delivered either to the lead tip or along the length of the lead.

Sheaths

Byrd dilator sheaths consist of two concentric tubes made of either TFE or the more rigid polypropylene that are passed over the lead and locking stylet. Controlled traction is delivered to the lead via the locking stylet while the dilator sheaths are advanced and rotated under fluoroscopic guidance, applying counterpressure at the site of fibrous adhesions (Figure 9.5). In this way, adherent fibrous tissue is disrupted or sheared away from the vessel wall. The sheaths are advanced to within a few millimeters of the lead tip–myocardium interface (Figure 9.6). At this point the blunt end of the outer sheath is fixed while countertraction is applied to the lead via the locking stylet. The sheath prevents invagination of the heart wall as tension on the lead tears the lead tip away from encapsulating scar tissue.

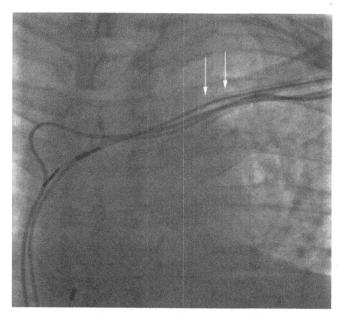

Figure 9.5 Radiograph showing extraction of a bipolar ventricular pacing lead by the superior approach. Arrows show the tips of the inner and outer Byrd dilator sheaths in the left subclavian vein. In this case, the only fibrous adhesions were at the proximal end of the lead and as these were freed, the lead retracted easily, shown here with its tip in the superior vena cava.

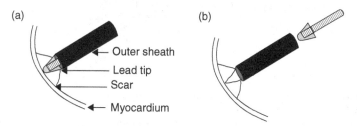

Figure 9.6 The principle of countertraction. The blunt end of the outer dilator sheath is fixed just proximal to the lead tip and traction is applied to the lead via the locking stylet. The outer sheath provides countertraction, preventing invagination and tearing of the thin right heart wall as the lead tip is avulsed from encapsulating fibrous tissue.

The Electrosurgical Dissection Sheath (EDS) incorporates a pair of bipolar diathermy electrodes at the beveled tip of the inner sheath to free adhesions (Figure 9.7). In theory, EDS may improve the success rate of complete lead removal by the superior approach, although published data are lacking.

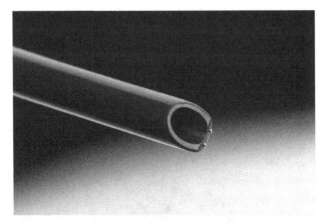

Figure 9.7 The Cook EDS. The sheath system resembles the Byrd dilator sheaths, with the addition of an electrode pair at the beveled tip of the inner sheath, allowing the delivery of bipolar diathermy in order to disrupt fibrous adhesions.

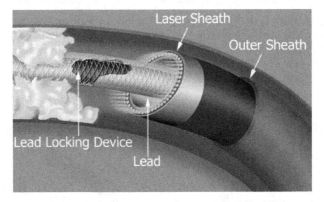

Figure 9.8 The Spectranetics laser sheath system comprises an inner and an outer sheath. The inner sheath contains a fiberoptic array delivering laser energy in a ring at the beveled tip of the sheath. A locking stylet is deployed within the inner conductor coil and the laser sheath is advanced over the lead. Laser energy is applied at the site of fibrous adhesions, freeing the lead.

An alternative system is the Spectranetics laser sheath, which can deliver laser energy in a ring at the tip of the sheath (Figure 9.8). Laser energy applied at tissue binding sites vaporizes intracellular water molecules thus dissolving the tissue. The tissue penetration depth of the laser beam is just $100\,\mu$m and therefore only tissue adherent to the lead is dissolved. In one randomized trial, the rate of successful lead extraction using a laser sheath was substantially higher than that using mechanical dilator sheaths alone.[4,5]

Inferior approach lead extraction

The workstation used to extract leads is introduced via the femoral vein opposite to the temporary pacing wire, preventing entanglement between the two.

Snares

After the permanent pacing leads have been freed at their proximal end, a stylet should be inserted and the leads advanced a short way. If the leads slide easily a Byrd femoral workstation should be used to extract the lead. If the leads do not slide easily, a needle's-eye snare should be used.[6] This is because the femoral workstation uses a relatively weak deflecting wire to pull the leads down from above (Figure 9.9). The leads are easily snared in the right atrium using this wire but large amounts of traction cannot be applied to the lead because the deflection wire breaks.

If the lead slides easily through the venous fibrous sheath it should be withdrawn to the inferior vena cava so that the proximal end of the lead

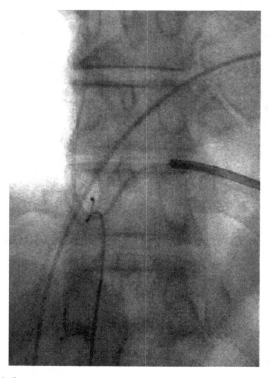

Figure 9.9 The deflection wire has been used to ensnare the body of a defibrillator lead in the right atrium. The lead was not tethered by fibrous adhesions proximally and the deflection wire was therefore used to pull the proximal end of the lead through.

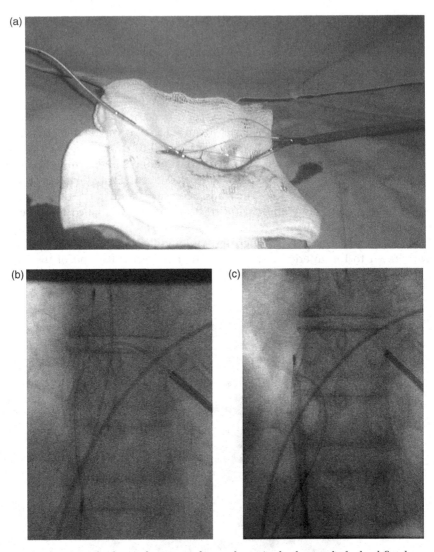

Figure 9.10 (a) A basket catheter may be used to grip the free end of a lead firmly. (b) Shows the open basket around the body of a defibrillator lead in the right atrium. (c) The inner sheath is advanced, closing the basket and gripping the lead firmly.

is hanging free. The basket that comes with the femoral workstation can then be advanced over the lead and closed so that the lead is captured (Figure 9.10).

The needle's-eye snare is not as easy to use when attempting to grasp the pacing leads but has the advantage of gripping the lead firmly (Figure 9.11).

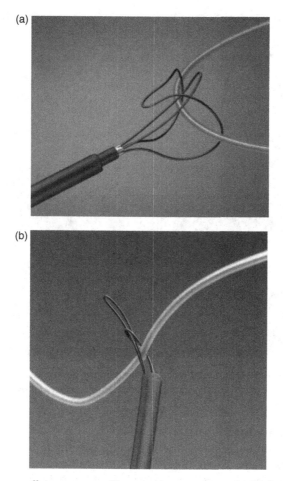

Figure 9.11 The needle's-eye snare. The outer loop ensnares the lead and the inner loop is then advanced from the sheath, trapping the lead body between the outer and inner loops (a). The sheath is then advanced, grasping the lead firmly between the outer and inner loops (b).

Sheaths

Once the lead is snared and pulled to the inferior cava, the 16 French outer sheath can then be advanced over the leads (Figure 9.12). The lead should be gently retracted as the 16 French sheath is advanced over the lead. For ventricular leads, the stiffness of the sheath will make it difficult to turn through the tricuspid valve, but will direct it away from the inferior wall of the right ventricle, a common point of fibrous tethering, and thus make it less likely to perforate the ventricle at this point. Once the sheath is ~1 cm away from the tip it should be held stationary and the lead pulled into the sheath (Figure 9.13).

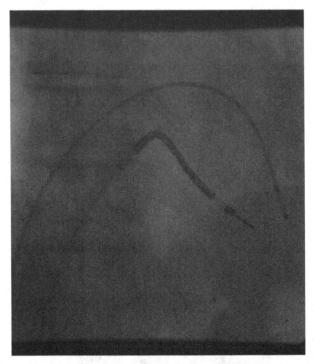

Figure 9.12 With the lead body firmly ensnared by the basket catheter, the blunt-ended outer sheath of the femoral workstation is advanced over the lead toward the apex of the right ventricle.

Access for new leads

The superior approach allows the extraction sheaths to be used to provide access for new leads. The femoral approach sheaths cannot be used for this purpose. It is, however, possible to wedge a 140 cm J-guidewire into a gap between the insulation and the coil at the proximal end of the leads to be extracted. This will be dragged through with the leads into the right atrium. This guidewire can then be used to introduce a sheath and new pacing leads into the cardiac chambers.[7,8]

Complications

The most serious complication of lead extraction is a tear of the great veins or cardiac wall resulting in intrapleural or pericardial bleeding, which may be catastrophic. Pulmonary embolism may occur with air, vegetations, or lead material. In one large series of 1684 patients undergoing laser-assisted extraction of chronically implanted pacemaker leads, serious complications as defined above occurred in 1.9% of patients with death in 0.8%. There is no convincing evidence of any difference in complication rate between mechanical (superior or inferior approach), electrosurgical, and laser sheath extraction.[5]

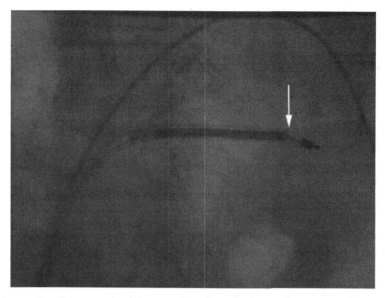

Figure 9.13 The outer sheath has been advanced to within 1 cm of the lead tip in the right ventricle (arrow). At this point the sheath is fixed and is used to deliver countertraction as the lead is withdrawn into the sheath, avulsing the lead tip from fibrous adhesions attaching it to the heart wall.

Traction on the right ventricle may prevent adequate filling and a low cardiac output. This is easily recognized with continuous arterial pressure monitoring and rapidly reversed by releasing the tension on the lead. Traction on the right ventricle invariably causes nonsustained arrhythmia and occasionally sustained ventricular tachycardia or fibrillation, although this usually terminates with release of tension on the lead.

Systemic sepsis is an unusual but serious complication following extraction of an infected system, and may be seen even when there has been no evidence of systemic infection before the procedure. This is presumably due to the release of toxins from the leads into the circulation during the procedure. The patient should be nursed in a high-dependency environment with close monitoring of temperature, blood pressure, arterial oxygen saturation, fluid intake, and urine output. A microbiologist should be involved early in the management and there is a strong case for the use of intravenous antibiotics for at least 48 hours following device extraction until it is clear that the patient is not going to develop systemic sepsis.

Indications for lead extraction

The indications for lead extraction can be considered in two groups: those where the risk of leaving the leads *in situ* clearly exceeds the risk of extraction and those where the decision to extract calls for careful consideration of the risks and benefits to the individual patient (Boxes 9.2 and 9.3).[9]

Box 9.2   Lead extraction mandatory

Septicemia
Endocarditis
Pocket infection
Erosion
Lead migration to dangerous position
Oversensing due to contact potentials between adjacent leads

Box 9.3   Lead extraction discretionary

Lead migration to safe position
Redundant leads
Potential danger from lead, for example, Accufix leads
Occlusion of great veins resulting in inability to pass new lead

---

The decision to extract may be influenced by other considerations including the experience of the operator, the duration of lead implantation, the type of lead(s) to be explanted, the age of the patient, and comorbidity such as terminal illness, coagulopathies and bleeding tendency, or a contraindication to thoracotomy.

Coronary sinus lead extraction

Until comparatively recently there have been few indications for the placement of a coronary sinus pacing or defibrillation lead and experience of lead extraction from the coronary sinus has been limited. The proven benefits of cardiac resynchronization therapy have led to a dramatic increase in the rate of coronary sinus lead implantation, and experience with coronary sinus lead extraction will inevitably follow. In the small reported series of coronary sinus lead extraction, conventional lead extraction techniques using locking stylets have been used, with or without a variety of sheaths. Care has been taken not to advance sheaths more than 1–2 cm into the coronary sinus to minimize the risk of trauma to the vein. There is some evidence from animal studies that fibrous adhesions do not develop between the wall of the coronary sinus and device leads to anything like the same extent as in the atrium or ventricle. This observation may help to explain why coronary sinus lead extraction has generally been successful and uncomplicated in reported series.[10]

Concluding remarks

Lead problems and device infections are never trivial and can result in important morbidity and even death. Treatment of device infection invariably involves complete device extraction, a procedure that requires skill and experience. Furthermore, management frequently involves difficult decisions about issues, such as the timing of device explantation, the need for temporary pacing, the duration of antibiotic therapy, and the timing of implantation of a new device. These patients should therefore always be referred to and managed in specialist pacing centers to ensure the best clinical outcome.

References

1 Byrd CL. Management of implant complications, in Ellenbogen KA, Kay GN, Wilkoff BL (eds). *Clinical cardiac pacing and defibrillation*. WB Saunders, Philadelphia, Pennsylvania, USA, 2000.

2 Miralles A, Moncada V, Chevez H *et al.* Pacemaker endocarditis: approach for lead extraction in endocarditis with large vegetations. *Ann Thorac Surg* 2001; 72: 2130–2.

3 Tyers GF. Similar indications but different methods: should there be a consensus or optimal lead extraction techniques? *Pacing Clin Electrophysiol* 2002; 25: 1019–22.

4 Wilkoff BL, Byrd CL, Love CJ *et al.* Pacemaker lead extraction with the laser sheath: results of the pacing lead extraction with the excimer sheath (PLEXES) trial. *J Am Coll Cardiol* 1999; 33: 1671–6.

5 Byrd CL, Wilkoff BL, Love CJ *et al.* Clinical study of the laser sheath for lead extraction: the total experience in the United States. *Pacing Clin Electrophysiol* 2002; 25: 804–8.

6 Klug D, Jarwe M, Messaoudene SA *et al.* Pacemaker lead extraction with the needle's eye snare for countertraction via a femoral approach. *Pacing Clin Electrophysiol* 2002; 25: 1023–8.

7 Staniforth AD, Schilling RJ. Reuse of occluded veins during permanent pacemaker lead extraction: a new indication for femoral lead extraction. *Indian Pacing Electrophysiol J* 2002; 2: 97.

8 Schilling R. Replacement of extracted permanent pacemaker or defibrillator leads by cannulation of veins using the femoral "drag-through" technique. *Heart* 2002; 87: 276–8.

9 Tyers GFO, Clark J, Wang Y *et al.* Coronary sinus lead extraction. *Pacing Clin Electrophysiol* 2003; 26: 524–6.

10 Bracke FA, Meijer A, van Gelder LM. Pacemaker lead complications: when is extraction appropriate and what can we learn from published data? *Heart* 2001; 85: 254–9.

Index

Note: Page numbers in *italics* represent figures; those in **bold** tables.